Chi Self-Massage

Chi Self-Massage

The Taoist Way of Rejuvenation

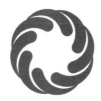

Mantak Chia

Destiny Books
Rochester, Vermont

Destiny Books
One Park Street
Rochester, Vermont 05767
www.DestinyBooks.com

Destiny Books is a division of Inner Traditions International

LIBRARY OF CONGRESS CATALOGING-IN-PUBLICATION DATA

Chia, Mantak, 1944–
    Chi self-massage : the Taoist way of rejuvenation / Mantak Chia.
[2nd ed.]
        p. cm.
    Includes index.
    ISBN-13: 978-1-59477-110-1
    ISBN-10: 1-59477-110-3
    1. Massage. 2. Medicine, Chinese. 3. Rejuvenation. I. Title.
    RA780.5.C48 2006
    615.8'22—dc22

                                                                2006004246

Printed and bound in Canada by Transcontinental Printing

10   9   8   7   6   5   4   3

Text design by Priscilla Baker
Text layout by Virginia Scott Bowman
This book was typeset in Janson Text with Present, Futura, Diotima, and Sho Roman
as the display typefaces

To send correspondence to the author of this book, mail a first-class letter to the
author c/o Inner Traditions • Bear & Company, One Park Street, Rochester, VT
05767, and we will forward the communication.

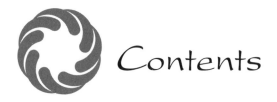

Contents

Acknowledgments

I thank foremost those Taoist masters who were kind enough to share their knowledge with me, never imagining it would eventually be taught to Westerners. I acknowledge special thanks to Dena Saxer for seeing the need for this book to be published and for her encouragement and hard work on the initial manuscript.

We wish to thank Nancy Yeilding and Vickie Trihy for editing this new edition of *Chi Self-Massage* and the following people who contributed to the first edition: Dena Saxer, for writing a portion of this book, especially the basic step-by-step instructions, and for choosing the title; Jo Ann Cutreria, for making so many contacts and working endlessly; Daniel Bobek, for long hours at the computer; John-Robert Zielinski and Adam Sacks for helping with the computer system; Helen Stites and Valerie Meszaros for editing and proofreading; and Gunther Weil, Rylin Malone, and many of my students, for their feedback. Special thanks are extended to Michael Winn, for general editing; to Juan Li, for spending many hours drawing and making illustrations of the body's internal functions and for his cover illustration; and to Felix Morrow, for his valuable advice and publication of the first edition.

Without my son, Max, the book would have been academic; for his gifts, my gratitude and love.

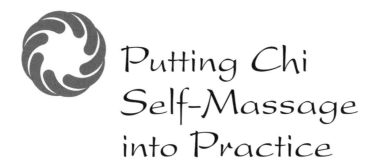

Putting Chi Self-Massage into Practice

The practices described in this book have been used successfully for thousands of years by Taoists trained by personal instruction. Readers should not undertake these practices without receiving personal transmission and training from a certified instructor of the Universal Tao, because certain practices described, if done improperly, may cause injury or result in health problems. This book is intended to supplement individual training by a Universal Tao instructor and to serve as a reference guide for the Universal Tao practices. Anyone who undertakes these practices on the basis of this book alone does so entirely at his or her own risk. Universal Tao instructors can be located at our Web sites: www.universal-tao.com and www.taoinstructors.org.

The meditations, practices, and techniques described herein are *not* intended to be used as an alternative or substitute for professional medical treatment and care. If a reader is suffering from a mental or emotional disorder, he or she should consult an appropriate professional health-care practitioner or therapist. Such problems should be corrected before one starts training.

This book does not attempt to give any medical diagnosis, treatment, prescription, or remedial recommendation in relation to any human disease, ailment, suffering, or physical condition whatsoever.

The Universal Tao and its staff and instructors cannot be responsible for the consequences of any practice or misuse of the information contained in this book. If the reader undertakes any exercise without strictly following the instructions, notes, and warnings, the responsibility must lie solely with the reader.

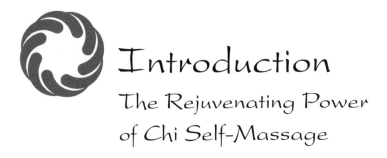

Introduction

The Rejuvenating Power of Chi Self-Massage

From ancient times to the present, Taoist masters have been remarkably youthful, appearing and functioning at least twenty years younger than their actual ages. One source of their vitality has been the practice of Taoist self-massage rejuvenation: using one's internal energy, or *chi*, to strengthen and rejuvenate the sense organs (eyes, ears, nose, tongue, skin) and the inner organs. These techniques are about five thousand years old and until now were closely guarded secrets passed on from one master to a small group of students. Even so, each master often knew only part of the practice. Based on my studies with a number of different Taoist masters, I have pieced together the entire method and organized the material into a logical routine. By practicing this routine daily, you can improve many aspects of your health, including your complexion, vision, hearing, sinuses, gums, teeth, tongue, and general stamina.

Chi Self-Massage rejuvenation works by clearing blockages from the meridians, or energy channels, of the various senses and vital organs. This is done by the unique Taoist practice of bringing energy, or chi, up from the sexual organs and anus to the face, hands, and senses, and then directing it to specific areas and organs of the body. When the organs—which are believed to store and generate positive and negative emotions—are energized by Chi Self-Massage, they become healthier, which, in turn, fosters positive changes in emotional and personal characteristics.

In my ten years of teaching this simple self-massage, I have seen many people use it to improve their emotional, personal, and social lives. One of my students, for example, had strong fears that easily brought on anger. This resulted in moodiness, irritability, and stomach pain. Naturally, someone who feels this way is unlikely to be very sociable or friendly. After a few weeks of practicing Chi Self-Massage, along with other techniques of Tao rejuvenation, this person's disposition improved, his moodiness decreased, and he became friendlier. He says that since he began studying with me, the greatest benefit has been to his family life, especially his relationship with his children. He no longer needs to use the alcohol he used to rely on to cover up his pain and forget his stress. His employer and coworkers have also noticed the change, and other workers have been encouraged to study the system.

Another person paid for one of her coworkers to study with us, wanting her coworker to find a way to better cope with stress on the job. She later told me that it was the best investment she had ever made, because she no longer had to contend with her coworker's emotional swings.

Chi Self-Massage is only one part of the Universal Tao system of self-development, which enables individuals to complete the harmonious evolution of their physical, mental, and spiritual bodies. Each of my books is an exposition of one important part of this system, and each sets forth a method of healing and life enrichment that can be studied and practiced by itself, if the reader so chooses. However, in the Taoist system each of these methods implies the others and they are best practiced in combination. Therefore I suggest that you also become familiar with the basic practices and exercises that form the foundation of Chi Self-Massage, particularly the Microcosmic Orbit and Inner Smile meditations outlined in the appendix and the Cosmic Healing Sounds outlined in my book *Taoist Cosmic Healing*. While the present book follows from all that has gone before it, you can begin with this book and learn from it the full range of Chi Self-Massage. Once you begin to practice and experience the benefits of this method of Taoist rejuvenation, however, you will no doubt wish to master the others, and you will find resources for further study at the Universl Tao Training Center (www.universal-tao.com, see page 108).

In the pages that follow you will find the techniques for raising and directing chi to bring its rejuvenating effects to all parts of your body, with chapters focusing specifically on the hands, head and sense organs, internal organs and glands, and knees and feet. Special attention is also given to the prevention and treatment of constipation, and the book concludes with comprehensive instructions for a daily practice to maintain abundant emotional and physical health.

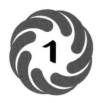

Preparing for Chi Self-Massage

A few simple guidelines should be followed to prepare yourself for doing Chi Self-Massage on any of the areas of the body shown in this book:

- Wait at least an hour after eating.
- To obtain the best results, try this practice immediately after doing the Inner Smile, the Microcosmic Orbit meditation, or the Six Healing Sounds (see my book *Taoist Cosmic Healing*).
- Sit comfortably on your sitting bones at the edge of a chair. Make sure that your legs are grounded. Those people who cannot get out of bed can practice the routine there.

RAISING THE CHI: PERINEUM POWER

In Tao rejuvenation the chi flow is very important. Without bringing chi circulation to the part of the body being massaged, it is just a simple, normal touch or massage. Raising the chi from the perineum region of the body and then directing it to where it is needed is a very important part of the preparation for Chi Self-Massage.

The perineum (Hui Yin) region includes the anus and sexual organs. The Chinese term Hui Yin means the "collection point of all the yin energy," or the lowest abdominal energy collection point. It is also known as the Gate of Life and Death. This gate lies between two other gates. The sexual organ, known as the Front Gate, is the big life-force opening from which energy can easily leak out and deplete the organ's function. The anus, known as the Back Gate, can also easily lose life-force when not sealed or closed tight. When these gates are open, the life-force and sexual energy can become "rivers of no return," flowing out and not recycling back. That is why Tao practices—especially the Tao Secrets of Love, Healing Love, Iron Shirt, and Chi Self-Massage—emphasize the perineum region's power to tighten, close, and draw the life-force back up the spine.

Organ Energy Is Connected with the Anus

The anus area itself is divided into five regions—middle, front, back, left, and right—each of which is closely linked to the chi of specific organs. By contracting the appropriate part of the anus as you prepare for and perform Chi Self-Massage, you can bring more chi to the organs and glands that need energy and the effects of the massage will increase (fig. 1.1).

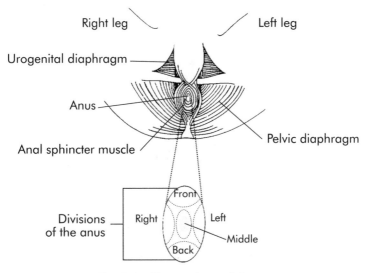

Fig. 1.1. **Five regions of the anus**

Middle Part of the Anus

The chi of the middle of the anus connects to the organs in the front part of the abdominal area: the vagina-uterus in women, the prostate gland in men, the aorta, the vena cava, the stomach, the heart, the thyroid and parathyroid glands, the pituitary gland, the pineal gland, and the top of the head (figs. 1.2 and 1.3).

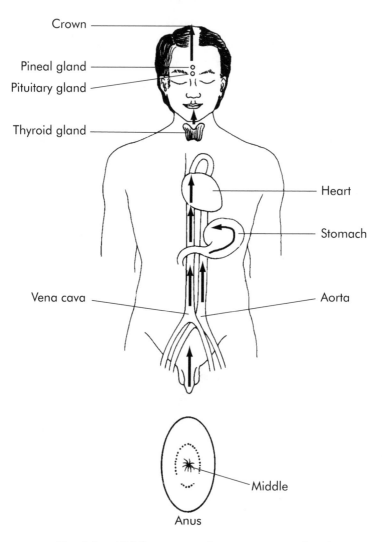

Fig. 1.2. Middle anus: male organ connections

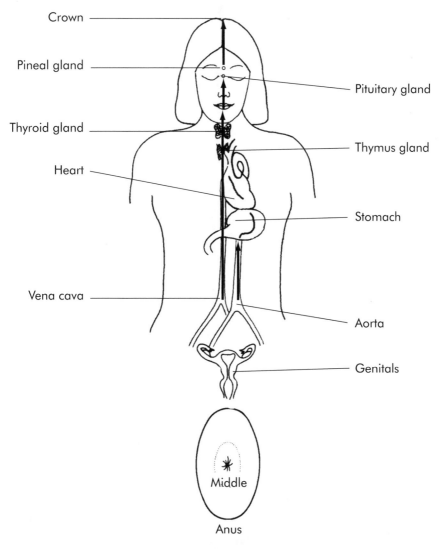

Crown

Pineal gland

Pituitary gland

Thyroid gland

Thymus gland

Heart

Stomach

Vena cava

Aorta

Genitals

Middle

Anus

Fig. 1.3. Middle anus: female organ connections

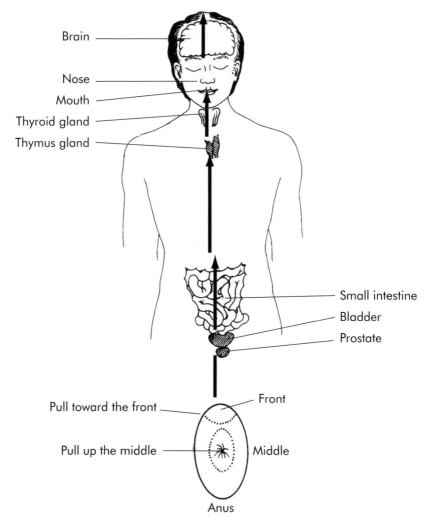

Fig. 1.4. Front anus: organ connections

Front Part of the Anus

The chi of the front of the anus connects to the prostate, bladder, small intestine, stomach, thymus gland, thyroid gland, and front part of the brain. When your Chi Self-Massage is directed to any of these organs, contract the anus and pull the middle part of the anus up toward the front (fig. 1.4).

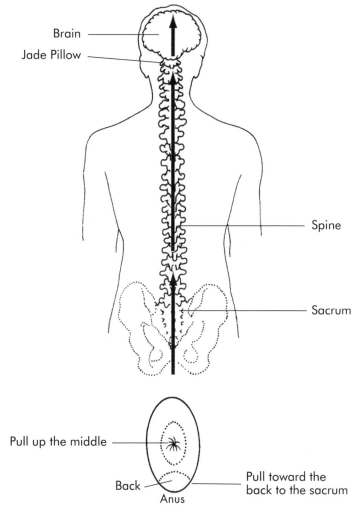

Brain

Jade Pillow

Spine

Sacrum

Pull up the middle

Back

Anus

Pull toward the
back to the sacrum

Fig. 1.5. Back anus: organ connections

Back Part of the Anus

The chi of the back of the anus is connected to the sacrum, the back of
the spine, and the cerebellum at the base of the skull, also known as the
Jade Pillow. When your Chi Self-Massage is directed to any of these
parts of the body, contract the anus and pull the middle part of the anus
up toward the back (fig. 1.5).

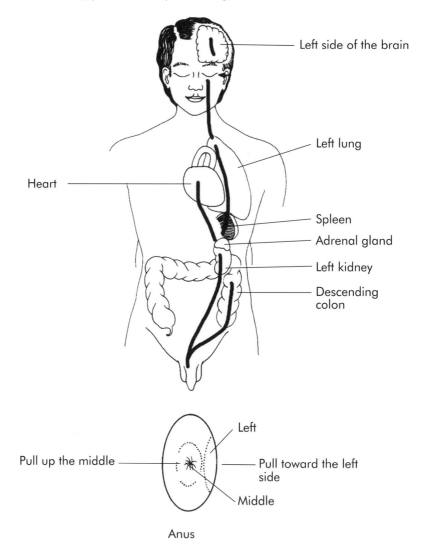

Left side of the brain

Left lung

Heart

Spleen

Adrenal gland

Left kidney

Descending colon

Left

Pull up the middle

Pull toward the left side

Middle

Anus

Fig. 1.6. Left anus: male organ connections

Left Part of the Anus

The chi of the left part of the anus is connected with the left ovary or left testicle, descending colon, left kidney, adrenal gland, spleen, left lung, and left hemisphere of the brain. When your Chi Self-Massage is directed to any of these organs, contract the anus and pull the middle part of the anus up toward the left side (figs. 1.6 and 1.7).

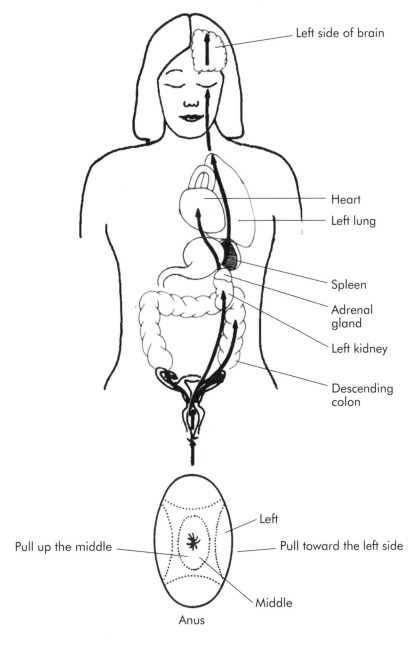

Left side of brain

Heart

Left lung

Spleen

Adrenal gland

Left kidney

Descending colon

Pull up the middle

Left

Pull toward the left side

Middle

Anus

Fig. 1.7. Left anus: female organ connections

Right Part of the Anus

The chi of the right part of the anus is connected to the right ovary or right testicle, ascending colon, right kidney, adrenal gland, liver, gallbladder, right lung, and right hemisphere of the brain. When your Chi Self-Massage is directed to any of these organs, contract the anus and pull the middle part of the anus up toward the right.

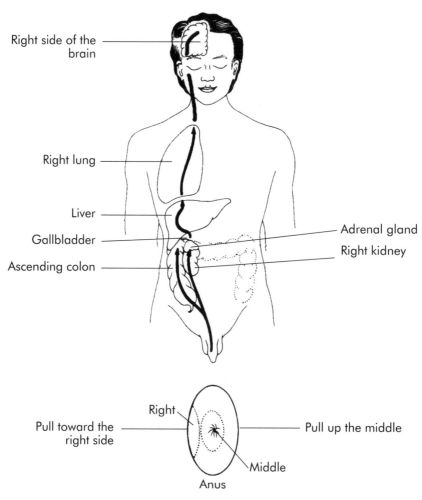

Fig. 1.8. Right anus: male organ connections

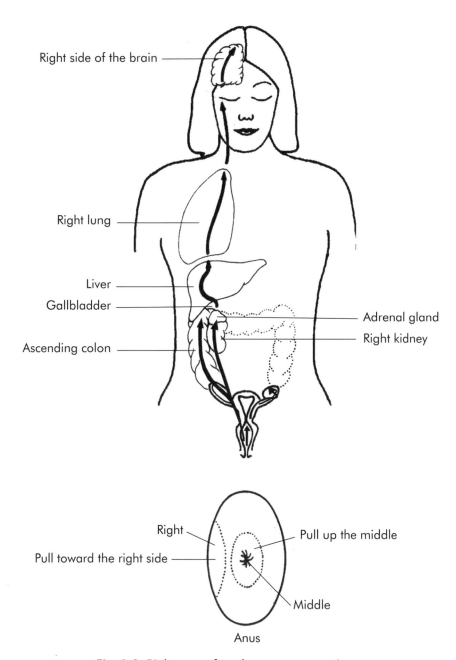

Right side of the brain

Right lung

Liver

Gallbladder

Ascending colon

Adrenal gland

Right kidney

Right

Pull up the middle

Pull toward the right side

Middle

Anus

Fig. 1.9. Right anus: female organ connections

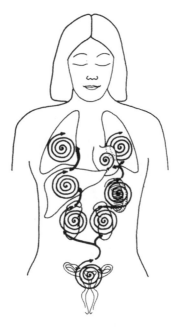

Fig. 1.10. Energy circling around the organs

Lifting the chi by contracting and lifting the correct part of the anus will direct it to circulate energy around the organs (fig. 1.10).

Beginning the Practice of Chi Self-Massage

Chi Self-Massage should always begin with raising the chi from the perineum to your hands, using the following method:

1. Inhale, contract your vagina or testicles, your buttocks, and also the part of the anus that corresponds to the location of the area to be massaged, that is, the front, back, right, left, middle, or entire anus. At first you may not be sensitive to these distinctions, but eventually you will be.
2. Hold your breath and hold the contractions, clench your teeth together, and press your tongue to the roof of your mouth as you rub your hands together vigorously.

3. Continue to rub your hands while holding your breath and contracting your anus. Feel your face getting hot. Then, mentally picture energy flowing to your hands.

4. When your face and hands are hot, exhale, breathe normally, direct your attention to the appropriate area, and begin to massage it. Smile and become aware of the part that is being massaged. Feel that the area is exceptionally warm and that energies are flowing.

5. Repeat this entire procedure for each area to be massaged or whenever your hands become cool. Your hands must always be very warm for self-massage, as cold hands will produce very little effect.

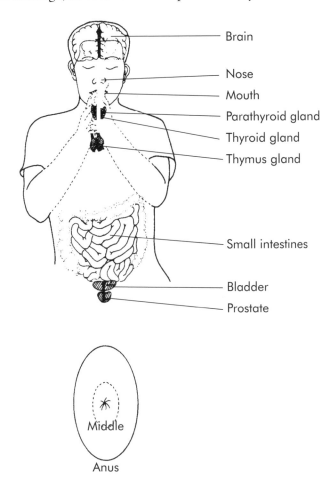

Fig. 1.11. Bringing chi to the hands

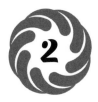

Healing Hands

Humans can build all kinds of sophisticated instruments because of the magnificence of their hands and fingers. Another higher function of the hands is the power of healing. The hands are particularly important in Chi Self-Massage not only because the massage of other parts of the body is done with the hands, but also because points on the hands correspond to various organs and functions of the body. Thus, massage of the major points on the hands stimulates and maintains the organs.

THE PALMS AND THE PERICARDIUM POINT

All major energies of chi join at the palms: they can receive energy, which then enters into the bone structure and into the major organs; the palms are also the place from which the life-force can be sent out to heal others or oneself.

At the center of the palm is the Pericardium point (P8), the main place of energy concentration and transmission (fig. 2.1).

CORRESPONDENCE POINTS ON THE HANDS

In the Universal Tao system, energy is understood to travel through the body along meridians, which connect the organs with the extremities. It is thus possible to correct energy blockages that are disrupting the

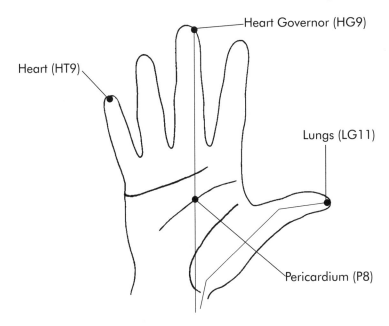

Fig. 2.1. Points on the palm and fingers

function of an organ by stimulating the connected point on the extremity. On the tips of the fingers, for example, there are termination points of the meridians for the Heart (HT9), Heart Governor (HG9), and Lungs (LG11) (fig. 2.1), as well as the Large Intestine (LI1) and Small Intestine (SI1) (fig. 2.2). The meridian known as the Triple Warmer connects the heart and head to a point (TW1) on the fingers.

The Large Intestine point on the back of the hand (LI4) is the major point used to control all the pain in the body, especially in the sense organs (eyes, ears, nose) and head (fig. 2.2).

The tips of the fingers have many tiny veins and arteries. When we get old and do not exercise enough, the chi does not flow well. This can affect blood circulation, and the veins and arteries will become hardened. The hands are the first places where cold is felt. If you want to warm up quickly, you have to warm the hands and feet first. The presence of the meridian points on the extremities also makes it possible to stimulate the organs by massaging the tips of the fingers (fig. 2.3).

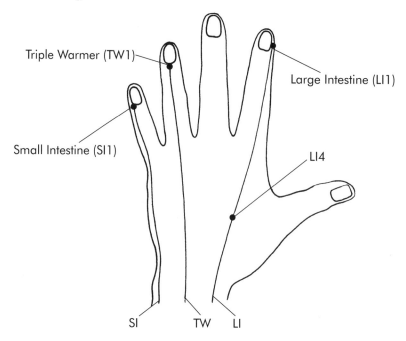

Triple Warmer (TW1)

Large Intestine (LI1)

Small Intestine (SI1)

LI4

SI   TW   LI

Fig. 2.2. Other major points on the hand and fingers

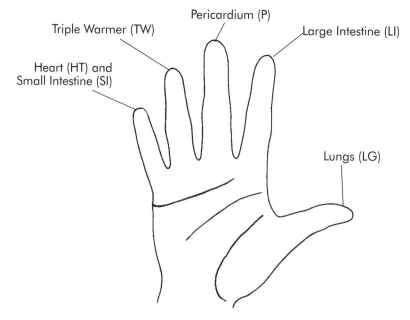

Pericardium (P)

Triple Warmer (TW)

Large Intestine (LI)

Heart (HT) and
Small Intestine (SI)

Lungs (LG)

Fig. 2.3. Fingertip massage stimulates corresponding organs

In addition to the meridian points on the hands, specific bodily functions can be seen as corresponding to the three major palm lines: the digestive and respiratory systems correspond to the Life Line; the nervous system corresponds to the Line of Intellect; and the circulatory and excretory systems correspond to the Line of Emotion (fig. 2.4).

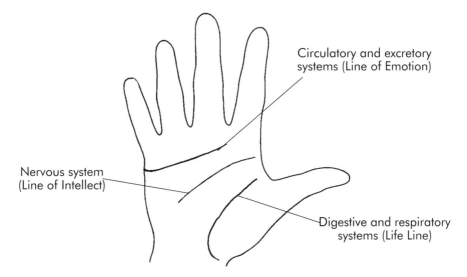

Fig. 2.4. Three major palm lines and corresponding functions

The organs that perform these functions can thus all be mapped on the hand, along with certain functions that correspond to specific sections and joints of the fingers (fig. 2.5).

Correspondence of the Fingers to Emotions and Elements

Each finger is also associated with one of the five elements and particular emotions:

- The thumb corresponds to the element earth, the stomach, and worry.
- The index finger corresponds to the element metal, the

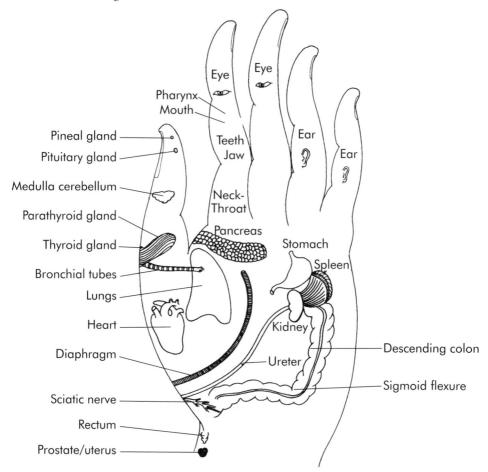

Fig. 2.5. Hands, fingers, joints, and their corresponding bodily functions

lungs and large intestine, and the emotions of sadness, grief, and depression.

- The middle finger corresponds to the element fire, the heart, small intestine, circulatory system, and respiratory system, and the emotions of impatience and hastiness.
- The ring finger corresponds to the wood element, the liver, gallbladder, and nervous system, and anger.
- The pinky finger corresponds to the water element, the kidneys, and fear.

HAND MASSAGE

Because of the many correspondences between the hands and various organs and functions, massaging the hands is a very effective way to increase the flow of chi throughout the body.

Performing Chi Hand Massage

The massage of the hands begins with the general preparation and raising of the chi to the hands outlined in chapter 1. The middle of the anus should be pulled up and toward the front. Then the following steps are performed.

1. Massage the Pericardium point (P8). Use the thumb to press the middle of the palm with a circular motion. Also massage the Pericardium point with the fingers cupped in the palm in a half-fist; the point is located where the tip of the middle finger rests (fig. 2.6).

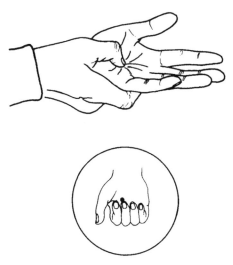

Fig. 2.6. **Massaging the pericardium point**

2. Massage the Large Intestine point known as the Hegu (LI4). Press the thumb around the point in a circular motion, particularly at

the base of the bone of the index finger. Find the pain point and massage it away (fig. 2.7).

3. Massage the major palm lines. Use the thumb to massage along the palm lines, particularly toward and along the thumb bone. When a lot of emotion is held inside, find the sore point and massage it with the thumb and fingers (fig. 2.8).

4. Massage the back of the hand, using the thumb to press along the

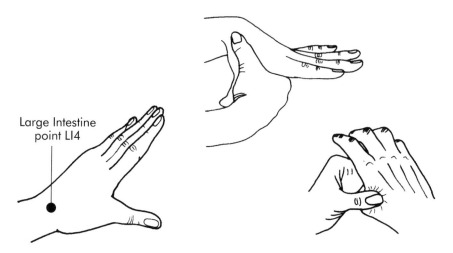

Large Intestine point LI4

Fig. 2.7. Massaging LI4

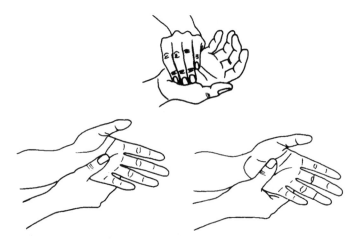

Fig. 2.8. Massaging the palm lines

bones. When you find a tender spot, take more time to work on it (fig. 2.9).

5. Massage the fingers. Remember to always rub your hands until warm. Use the right hand's thumb and forefinger to stimulate the points shown on each finger of the left hand, then do the same for the right hand with the thumb and forefinger of the left (fig. 2.10).

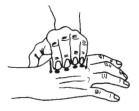

Fig. 2.9. Massaging the back of the hand

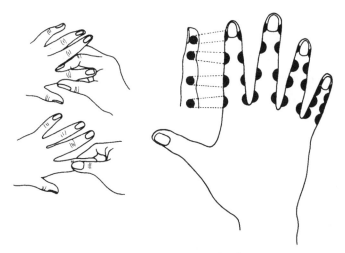

Fig. 2.10. Massaging the fingers

🌀 Wrapping the Fingers

Wrapping a finger calms its related emotion (fig. 2.11). Wrap the fingers of the right hand around the left thumb, and then, one by one, squeeze, hold, and release each finger on the left hand three to six

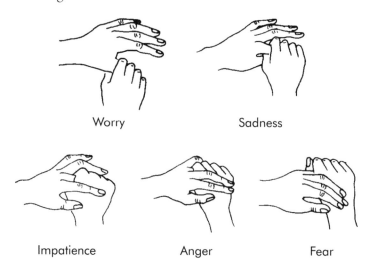

Worry   Sadness

Impatience   Anger   Fear

Fig. 2.11. Wrapping the fingers to control emotions

times. Then use the fingers of the left hand to wrap the thumb and fingers of the right hand, one by one.

This method can be used to gain control of your negative emotions at any time. If, for example, you start to get angry, try to wrap your ring finger a few times to reduce your anger. If you are frightened or fearful, wrap your fingers around your little fingers, starting with the left side and moving to the right side. This can be a great help when you are in a difficult situation, such as talking before a group of people, going to an interview, or meeting important people. Practicing the Heart and Kidney Sounds in conjunction with the finger wrapping may also help.

This technique can also be used to help overcome addiction to tobacco, drugs, or alcohol. The toxic elements found in these substances settle in the organs and nervous system, stimulating them into over-activity, quickly causing the user to feel "high." But when the effect wears off, the person will start to feel very low energy, becoming emotional and nervous. To calm down in such a situation, the Inner Smile and Microcosmic Orbit circulation can be used in combination with holding the fingers, especially the ring finger. Repeated practice of this technique will give the disciple the strength and power to clean out the accumulated toxins in the system, and to eliminate bad habits.

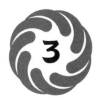

Head, Neck, and Shoulders

The head is the place where all the nerves are seated and is the central control of the whole system, so when Chi Self-Massage is done on the head, the whole nervous system can be strengthened. In addition, the massage of each specific area of the head has particular beneficial effects.

SKULL MASSAGE

The massage of the skull is particularly helpful for relieving headaches, nervousness, and an imbalance of energy in the brain. Many young people today experience extreme nervousness, which causes insomnia, appetite loss, increased heartbeat, breathing difficulties, tiredness, laziness, and so on. While these symptoms may not initially be signs of a disease, when they continue over a long period of time, they greatly affect a person's work efficiency and may gradually be considered mental disease.

The glands, senses, and organs can be weakened when the chi in the brain is not balanced. During the massage of the skull, the tongue is placed on the roof of the mouth and the eyes are moved up to the left and then across to the right; this technique stimulates the energy from left to right in order to balance the left and right hemispheres of the brain.

The skull massage also increases blood circulation in the head and the supply of nutrition to the scalp and hair. Many of our students who practice it regularly have had the experience of thinning hair being replaced by more vigorous growth, or white hair being replaced by black hair. The hair also grows softer. The effect of the head massage can be enhanced by brushing the hair twenty-five to fifty times in the morning and at night with a good brush. Of course, if you practice this, you should be careful not to scratch your scalp, which might result in a headache or sense of pain.

Performing Skull Massage

The skull massage, like all aspects of Chi Self-Massage, begins with the general preparation and raising of the chi to the hands and face as outlined in chapter 1. The part of the anus to be contracted is the middle. Then the following steps are performed.

1. Place your tongue on the roof of your mouth and move your eyes up to the left and then across to the right while doing the other steps.
2. Massage the Crown point, which is located in the center of the crown (in the fontanel area of an infant's skull there may still be a slight depression at this point) (fig. 3.1). The Crown point is the junction of one hundred channels through which the energy of the body passes. This area should be massaged with both middle fingers. This will relieve dizziness and headaches, which result from too much energy in the head. It also relieves high blood pressure and stimulates the nervous system.
3. Lightly hit your skull with the knuckles of both hands, knocking all around the head (fig. 3.2). Knocking the head lightly can help to clear your head, eliminate stubbornness, and make your thinking sharper. This knocking of the head helps to release the pressures caused by today's fast-moving life of advanced technology and the feeling of always having to keep up. It can be especially helpful for students

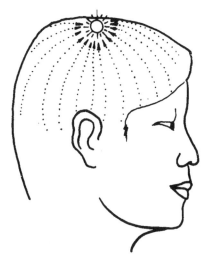

Fig. 3.1. Crown point, junction of one hundred energy channels

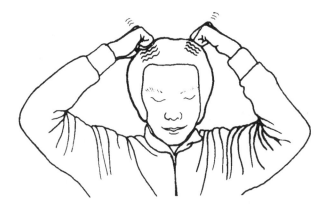

Fig. 3.2. Knocking the head

who feel a great deal of stress about keeping up with their studies. When too much pressure accumulates in their heads, they are unable to think clearly, which leads to worry, fear, sadness, and sometimes suicide. The simple knocking of the head can release pressure and stress that accumulate there and prevent such dire results.

4. Massage your scalp. Hold your breath for some time before starting in order to increase the chi flow to the head. Then, using both hands like a comb, press hard and slowly massage the scalp straight

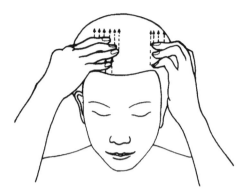

Fig. 3.3. Massaging the scalp

back from the hairline to the base of the skull (fig. 3.3). As you do this, mentally direct your energy from the back of the skull to your feet. Repeat six to nine times. In any places where you feel pain, continue to massage until the pain goes away.

5. Massage the crest, the edge at the base of the skull (fig.3.4). Many meridians pass through the crest to join in the skull, particularly at the crown of the head. In Tao tradition the crest is called the Pool of Wind, because it tends to collect the negative energy known as the "evil wind," the major cause of all the pain in the senses. Moving your thumbs up and down as shown in figure 3.5, massage the crest, particularly the points known as Fengchi, until you feel no pain there. This will help you reduce headaches and eye aches and will enhance vision.

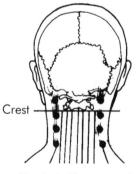

Fig. 3.4. The crest, the edge of the skull

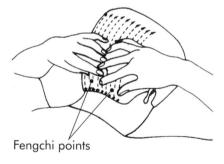

Fig. 3.5. Massage of the crest

FACE MASSAGE

The appearance of your face forms the first impression that is imprinted in other people's minds. Good chi circulation provides the face with attractive personal energy. Massaging your face with chi causes the skin to glow brightly and appear more youthful: it is a far more effective beauty treatment than the most expensive cream or cosmetic.

When you are massaging your face, it is helpful to keep in mind the many muscles that are found there (fig. 3.6).

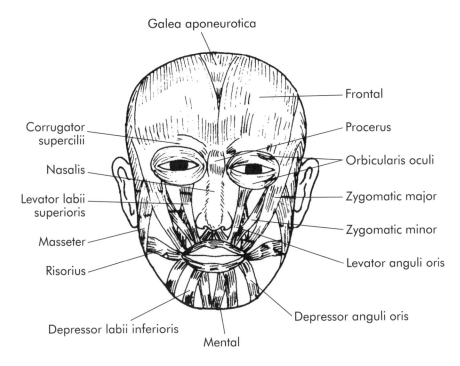

Fig. 3.6. Facial muscles

Many meridians pass through or end at the face, connecting many organs and areas of the body with areas of the face. Two different mappings indicate the great number of correspondences to be found on the face (figs. 3.7 and 3.8). When the meridians are blocked, they result in a reduced flow of chi and poor circulation, interfering with the proper functioning of the connected parts. Chi Self-Massage of the face

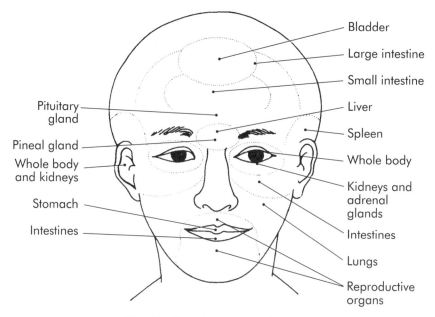

Fig. 3.7. Facial correspondences

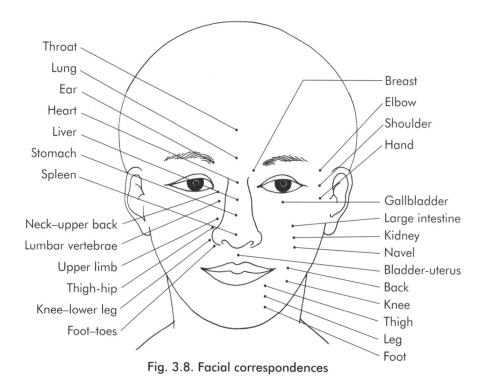

Fig. 3.8. Facial correspondences

removes blockages and enhances the health of the organs and other areas.

Performing Chi Face Massage

The massage of the face begins with the general preparation and raising of the chi to the hands and face as outlined in chapter 1. The part of the anus to be contracted is the middle and front. Then the following steps are performed.

1. Wipe your forehead from one side to the other six to nine times, using alternate hands (fig. 3.9).

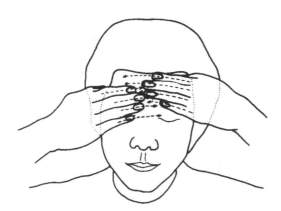

Fig. 3.9. Wiping the forehead

2. Wipe the middle section of the face, from the eyebrows to the tip of your nose. Using alternate hands, wipe from one side to the other and then up and down (fig. 3.10).
3. Wipe the lower section of the face, below the nose to your chin. Using alternate hands, wipe from one side to the other and then up and down.
4. Repeat the procedure for bringing energy to your hands. Inhale, cover your whole face with your palms and massage it (fig. 3.11). Use an upward motion to reduce wrinkles. Exhale and relax your

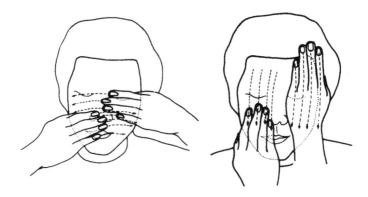

Fig. 3.10. Wiping the mid-face

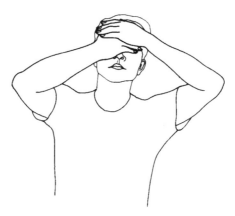

Fig. 3.11. Massaging the whole face

face. Rest and smile to your face until you can feel it tingle with warmth.

5. Massage the middle of your forehead, from the center to the temple, using the second joint of your index fingers (fig. 3.12).

6. Massage the temples and forehead with the knuckles of your index fingers. Massage the temples in a circular motion, first clockwise, then counterclockwise. Then rub from the middle of the forehead all the way to the temples ten to twenty times, using the same circular motions (fig. 3.13). These exercises will reduce headaches in the front of the head and in the temples. Find any painful point and massage it until the pain is gone.

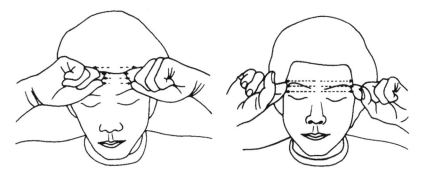

Fig. 3.12. Massaging the mid-forehead

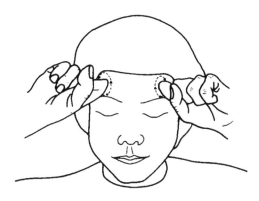

Fig. 3.13. Massaging the temples and forehead

EYE MASSAGE

The eyes are the doorways to the soul (fig. 3.14). They are connected to the entire nervous system, which gives them a special importance. In Taoism the eyes are regarded as yang energy that guides all chi flow in the body.

The different areas of the eyes correspond to different organs of the body (fig. 3.15), so they reveal the health of your entire body: you can tell which organs are weak or toxic by looking at your eyes. Nowadays people use their eyes much more than in the past to read, watch

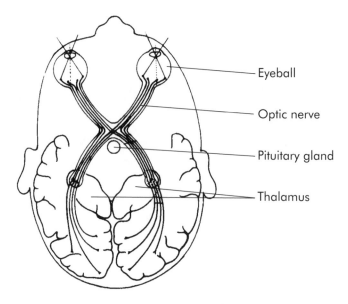

Fig. 3.14. Eyes, doorways to the soul

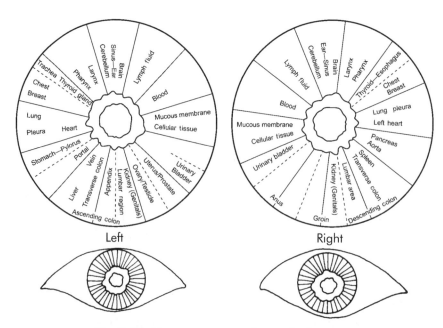

Fig. 3.15. Organ correspondences in the eyes

television, and work with computers, other electronic devices, and microscopes. This strains them a great deal and allows much of the energy of the connected organs to be drained out. Massaging the eyes will reenergize the vital organs.

Performing Eye Massage

Begin with the procedure for bringing energy to the hands and face, contracting the middle, left, and right sides of the anus. When your hands and face are hot, direct the chi to both eyes until you feel them filled with energy.

1. Close your eyes. Use your fingertips to gently massage your eyeballs through your closed eyelids, six to nine times clockwise, then six to nine times counterclockwise. Then gently massage the area around the lids the same number of times (fig. 3.16). Be aware of painful spots and massage those places until the pain goes away. Pay special attention to the inner and outer corners of the eyes. Massaging these points of the Gall Bladder meridian will relieve

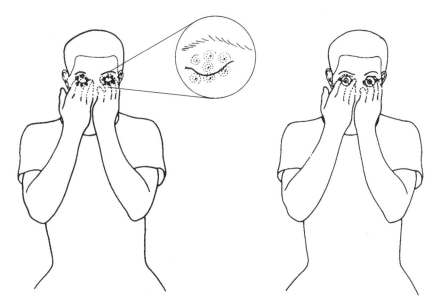

Fig. 3.16. Massaging the eyeballs and around the lids

eye ailments. However, when rubbing near the corners of the eyes, do not rub too hard, because you can make the corners of the eyes droop down. Finish with rubbing the corners of the eyes upward.

2. Pull up the eyelids to increase the fluid. Use the thumb and index finger to gently pinch and pull up the eyelids, then release them. Do this six to nine times (fig. 3.17).

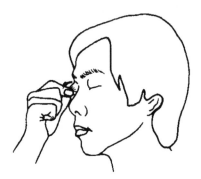

Fig. 3.17. Pulling up the eyelids

3. Massage the eye sockets by bending your index fingers and using the lower section to rub the upper and lower bones of the eye sockets six to nine times (fig. 3.18).

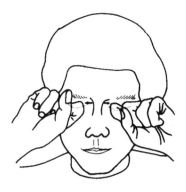

Fig. 3.18. Massaging the eye sockets

4. The next step is to get a tear out of your eyes, which will strengthen them. Hold an index finger up about eight inches from your eyes (or put a dot on the wall five to six feet away from you). Stare at it intently without blinking until you feel like a fire is burning in your eyes (fig. 3.19). The Taoists believe that this technique burns the toxins out of the body through the eyes.

5. Bring chi to your eyes by rubbing your hands until they are warm, then closing your eyes and covering your eye sockets with your palms. Feel the chi from the hands being absorbed into the eyes. Rotate your eyes six to nine times, first in a clockwise direction, then counterclockwise (fig. 3.20).

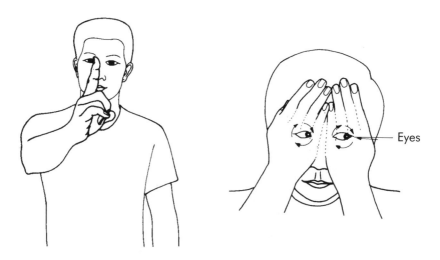

Fig. 3.19. Getting a tear out   Fig. 3.20. Absorbing chi into the eyes

EYEBALL EXERCISE

The eyes have many muscles that we typically do not exercise very much. This causes them to become weak, contributing to poor eyesight. In addition, the eyes are closely connected with certain organs and nerves (fig. 3.21). Exercising the eyeballs not only is the best exercise for the eye muscles but also will exercise these linked areas by putting pressure on them:

- Contracting the middle of the eyeballs strengthens the back of the eye muscles and the inner ear.
- Moving the eyeballs upward by looking toward the crown strengthens the upper eye muscles and stimulates the pituitary and pineal glands.
- Moving the eyeballs from side to side strengthens the side eye muscles as well as the ear canals, eardrums, tear ducts, and nose.
- Moving the eyes downward strengthens the lower eye muscles as well as the lower parts of the ear canals and the nervous system.

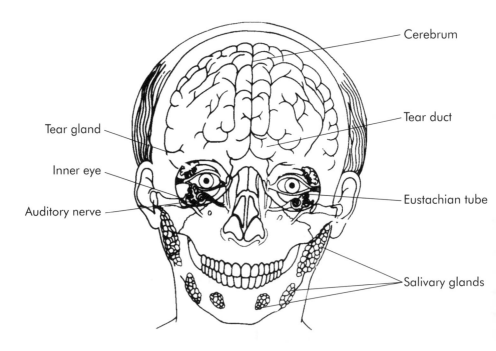

Fig. 3.21. Nerves, organs, and glands near the eyes

Performing the Eyeball Exercise

This exercise begins with closing the eyes and becoming aware of them (fig. 3.22).

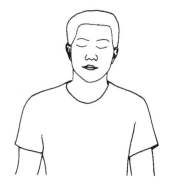

Fig. 3.22. Awareness of the eyes

With the eyes still closed, cup your palms over them, inhale, and contract the sexual organ and the part of the anus as directed, while looking straight ahead, to the left, above, to the right, and below (fig. 3.23).

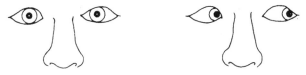

(1) Pressing into the inner ear

(2) Left eye pressing into the ear canal; right eye pressing into the eustachian tube

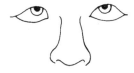

(3) Pressing into the pituitary gland

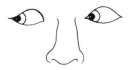

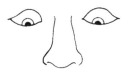

(4) Right eye pressing into the ear canal; left eye pressing into the eustachian tube

(5) Pressing into the eustachian tube

Fig. 3.23. Moving the eyes

1. Contract the middle of the anus, and pull the eyeballs back into their sockets.
2. Contract the left side of the anus and the left sides of the eyeballs.
3. Contract the front of the anus and the tops of the eyeballs.
4. Contract the right side of the anus and the right sides of the eyeballs.
5. Contract the back of the anus and the bottoms of the eyeballs.

STARING PRACTICE

If you have difficulty maintaining eye contact when you are talking with someone because you feel nervous and frightened, this can be caused by weakness of the gallbladder and kidneys. You may also experience that your voice becomes very low and hard to hear. To improve this, you can use the Inner Smile, Six Healing Sounds, and Chi Self-Massage as described above, plus the practice of staring.

To perform the practice of staring, look at your face in a mirror for two to five minutes each day for the first week. After ten days you can begin to stare at your eyes and increase your confidence by looking at your irises. Gradually you will lose the fear of looking into other people's eyes.

NOSE MASSAGE

The nose has several important functions, including breathing, temperature regulation, and smell. It is the first place into which the breath of life enters. A healthy nose helps us to have good chi throughout the body. When we breathe properly through the nose and not through the mouth, it filters out dirt, preventing it from reaching the lungs. The nose also regulates the temperature of the air being breathed in: when the air is too cold, the nose warms it up first.

The nose has three meridians running through it: the Large Intestine, the Stomach, and the Governor or Back Channel. In China just a few needles inserted in the nose serve as a general anesthetic for any part of the body to be operated on.

A weak or infected nose blocks the flow of chi and allows a lot of mucus to leak into the sinuses. It interferes with the sense of smell and may also affect the voice, interfering with speaking and singing. When the nose is unable to properly perform its temperature-regulating action, extreme temperatures make us susceptible to colds and other upper respiratory illnesses and can even injure the lungs. An unhealthy nose also affects the personality, making a person less attractive to other people.

Rubbing and massaging the nose opens the passages, increases the chi, strengthens the temperature regulator, and improves circulation around the nose, all of which contribute to the rare occurrence of colds in practitioners of this Tao rejuvenation system. Nose massage also stimulates the large intestine and the stomach and increases hormone secretion.

Performing Nose Massage

Repeat the procedure for bringing energy to your hands, contracting the front part of the anus.

1. Widen the nostrils using the thumb and index finger (fig. 3.24). Stick them into the nostrils and move them to the left and the right

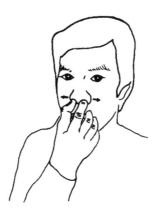

Fig. 3.24. Widening the nostrils

and up and down ten to twenty times. This will increase the passage of air into the lungs. It can also help remedy sinus problems and correct problems with the sense of smell.

2. Use your thumb and index finger to massage the bridge of your nose by repeatedly pinching it. As you do this, inhale slowly and imagine you are breathing in clean air; exhale slowly and imagine you are exhaling dirty air. Do this nine to thirty-six times (fig. 3.25). This is effective for blocked sinuses.

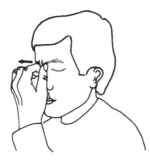

Fig. 3.25. Massaging the bridge

3. To massage your mid-nose, place your thumb on one side and third finger on the other, right on the bone that runs perpendicular to the nose. Place your index finger on the bridge (fig. 3.26). Inhale and press in gently. Exhale and relax. Feel and absorb the heat from your fingers into the nose. This can increase your concentration and calm your mind.

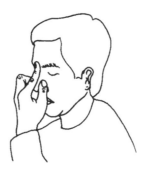

Fig. 3.26. Massaging the mid-nose

4. Use your index fingers to massage up and down the sides of the nose nine to thirty-six times (fig. 3.27). Do this slowly, gradually increasing the pressure. Be careful not to press too hard in the beginning because the sensitive tissues there are very tender and easily infected. Rub the sides of your nose up and down until you feel warm. This should be done every morning when you get up and will be especially helpful in cold weather. It also helps blocked sinuses and stuffy noses.

5. Massage the lower nose by vigorously rubbing an index finger back and forth right under it at a right angle to the nose (fig. 3.28). Massage slowly, and gradually increase the pressure when you are sure you will not hurt yourself. This helps blocked sinuses and stuffy, runny noses.

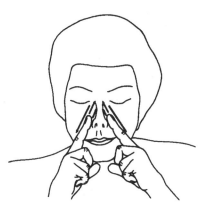

Fig. 3.27. Massaging the sides of the nose

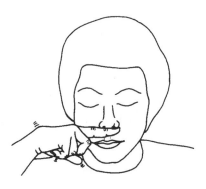

Fig. 3.28. Massaging the lower nose

EAR MASSAGE

In addition to being the organs of hearing, the ears are acupuncture maps of the whole body, containing 120 points. Many acupuncturists now use only the ear points to cure many ailments as well as for weight control. Massage of the ears can stimulate those points as well as prevent the hearing loss that occurs gradually as we age.

Performing Ear Massage

Repeat the method for bringing energy to the hands, contracting the left and right sides of the anus.

1. Make a space between your index and middle fingers and simultaneously rub in front and in back of the ears (fig. 3.29a).
2. Rub the ear shells with all of your fingers. This will stimulate the autonomic nervous system and warm up your whole body, especially in cold weather (fig. 3.29b).
3. Using your thumb and index finger, pull down on the ear lobes (fig. 3.29c).

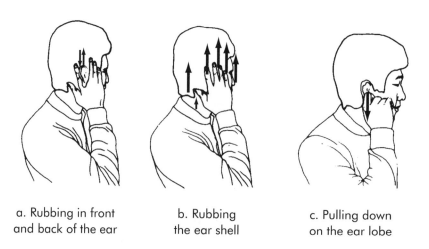

a. Rubbing in front and back of the ear

b. Rubbing the ear shell

c. Pulling down on the ear lobe

Fig. 3.29. Rubbing the ear

EARDRUM EXERCISES

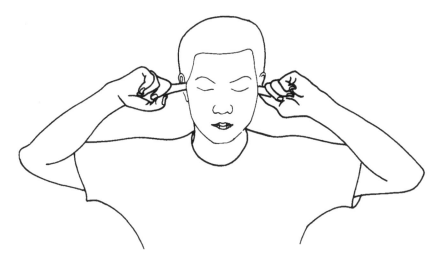 Outer Eardrum Exercise

To exercise the outer eardrum, repeat the method for bringing energy to the hands, contracting the left and right sides of the anus.

1. Inhale and then exhale completely.
2. Put your index fingers in your ears; it should feel as if there is a vacuum in the ears. If it does not, then exhale more.
3. Move your index fingers back and forth six to nine times at your own pace until you can feel that the eardrums are gently flexing back and forth, then pull out your fingers with a quick movement (fig. 3.30). You should hear a "pop" sound, and you will feel that you can hear better and that your mind is clearer.

Please note that this exercise should be done gently to avoid injury to the eardrums. The "popping" sound is made by the sudden release of the suction created by holding the breath and moving the fingers in the ears.

Fig. 3.30. Outer eardrum exercise

⟁ Inner Eardrum Exercises

The inside of the inner ear, being inaccessible, is usually not exercised and grows weaker with age (fig. 3.31). These two exercises use air pressure and vibrations to strengthen the inner ear.

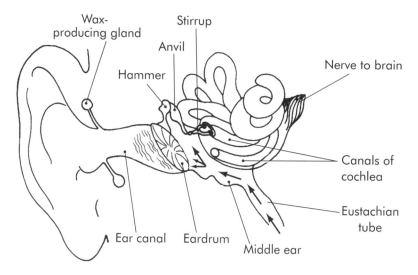

Fig. 3.31. Diagram of inner eardrum

Both inner ear exercises should begin with the method for bringing energy to the hands, contracting the left and right sides of the anus. The ear canals, the nose canal, and the mouth are connected, so the first exercise uses the pressure that builds in the lungs to add pressure to the inner eardrums by bringing it back up to the mouth (fig. 3.32).

1. Blowing exercise: First inhale and fill your lungs and nasal cavity with air, then close your mouth and pinch your nostrils shut with your index finger and thumb. Slowly blow the air out through your closed nostrils and then swallow air. You should feel your eardrums popping, as they often do with a change in altitude. Repeat two or three times (fig. 3.32). This exercise must be done gently to get the most benefit. Especially avoid blowing too hard, as that can injure the eardrums.

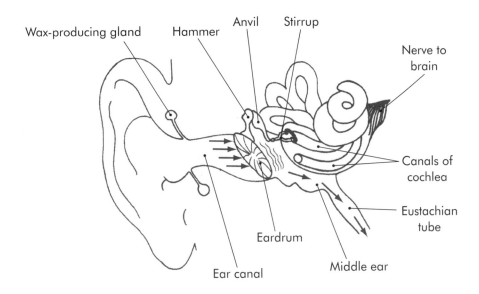

Wax-producing gland   Hammer   Anvil   Stirrup   Nerve to brain   Canals of cochlea   Eustachian tube   Middle ear   Eardrum   Ear canal

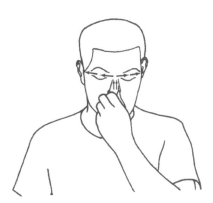

Fig. 3.32. Inner eardrum exercise

2. Vibration Exercise: Cover your ears with your palms, fingers pointing toward the back of your head. In this position, flick your index fingers against your third fingers so that the index fingers drum on the lower edge (occipital bone) of the skull (fig. 3.33). This will sound quite loud as it impacts the eardrum. The flicking of the finger to hit the bones vibrates and stimulates the nervous system, the ears, and the inner ears' mechanism. Repeat nine or

more times. The activity of the ear will be balanced and the mastoid sinus improved by this exercise.

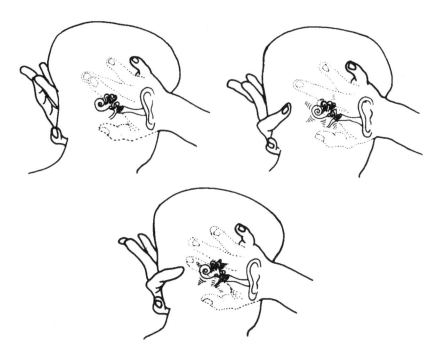

Fig. 3.33. Flicking the index fingers against the skull

MOUTH MASSAGE

The flow of energy in the body and the expression of the face are the main attractive powers of a person. Looking cheerful, delightful, attractive, and happy depends very much on the appearance of the corners of the mouth. Stress, depression, and sadness can depress the energy system and loosen the muscles of the mouth, causing the corners of the mouth to droop. No one likes to look at a sad face or a depressed face; it makes other people feel sad and depressed, too. Massaging the mouth muscles up will help to lift the corners of the mouth. This can be combined with the Inner Smile to build up attractive energy.

🌀 Beautify the Mouth Massage

Begin with the procedure for bringing energy to your hands and face.

Using the thumb and the index finger of the right hand, touch both corners of the mouth and feel the chi from the thumb and index finger pass to the corners of the mouth. Slowly press and push up about one inch and release; start again at the corners, pressing up ten to twenty times each day (fig. 3.34).

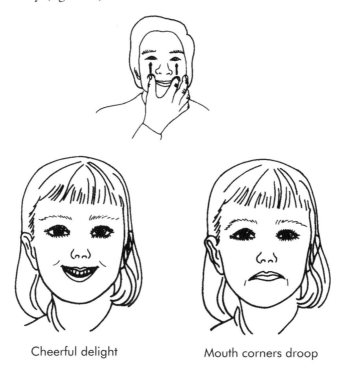

Cheerful delight   Mouth corners droop

Fig. 3.34. Beautify the mouth massage

GUMS, TONGUE, AND TEETH MASSAGE AND EXERCISES

Teeth are the excess energy of the bones, and when the teeth get stronger, so do the bones. Healthy teeth require healthy gums as their foundation.

The tongue is the opening of the heart, and both are made of similar tissue. The tongue corresponds to several internal organs, so a healthy and clean tongue will strengthen the organs, especially the heart (figs. 3.35 and 3.36). The saliva in the mouth is an essential form of energy that lubricates the organs and digestive system. Chi Self-Massage includes massage and exercises to strengthen the teeth, tongue, and gums.

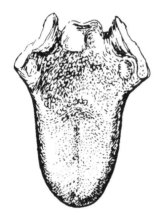

Fig. 3.35. Tongue

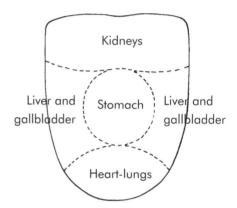

Fig. 3.36. Tongue parts and corresponding organs

Performing Gum Massage

Begin with the procedure for bringing energy to the hands and face, contracting the middle of the anus.

1. Open your mouth and stretch your lips tautly over your teeth. Use three fingertips (index, middle, and ring fingers) to tap the skin around the upper and lower gums until you feel warmth in the area (fig. 3.37).
2. Massage your upper and lower gums with your tongue (fig. 3.37).

Performing Tongue Massage

Begin with the procedure for bringing energy to the hands and face, contracting the middle of the anus.

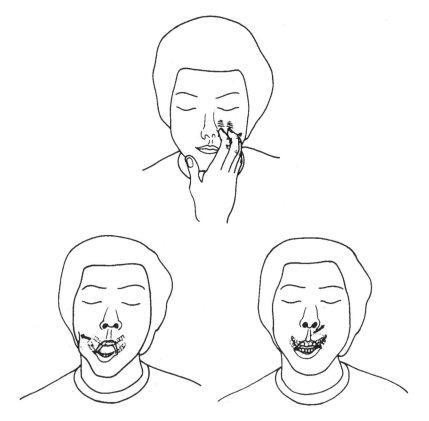

Fig. 3.37. Hitting the gums and tongue massage of the gums

Massage your tongue with a tongue depressor or a clean finger (fig. 3.38). Find the painful spots and massage there until the pain goes away.

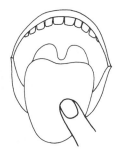

Fig. 3.38. Massaging the tongue

⟲ Tongue Exercises

These exercises will help to strengthen the throat and the tongue and to improve the clarity of speech and bad breath.

1. Sit erect with your hands on your knees, palms down.
2. Exhale and straighten your arms, spreading your fingers apart and keeping your hands on your knees.
3. Open your mouth as wide as possible and thrust your tongue out and down toward your throat. With your tongue out as far possible, gaze at the tip of your nose. Your whole body should be tense. Hold your breath for as long as you feel comfortable.
4. Relax with inhalation and regulate your breath.
5. Inhale, then exhale as you press your tongue out and down as far as you can. Follow with pulling the tongue in and curling it. Press your tongue to the roof of your mouth as hard as you can, while simultaneously contracting the middle of the anus and the esophagus to help the tongue (fig. 3.39). With practice you will learn how to use the inside force, the force from the organs, to press your tongue up. Even though the tongue has no bones to exert force, you will still be able to exercise the tongue well.

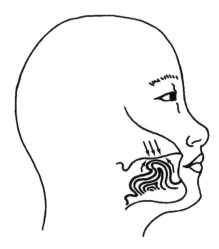

Fig. 3.39. Pressing the tongue to the roof of the mouth

6. Move your tongue and mouth to create a lot of saliva. Without curling your tongue, press it tightly against the palate while holding the saliva in your mouth. Continuing to press your tongue to the roof of your mouth, tighten your neck muscles and swallow the saliva quickly with a hard gulp, sending the saliva down the esophagus to your stomach. This lubricates the digestive glands and organs.

🌀 Teeth Exercises

1. Relax your lips. Click the teeth together lightly (fig. 3.40) and then clench them hard (fig. 3.41) as you inhale and pull up the middle of the anus. Do this six to nine times.

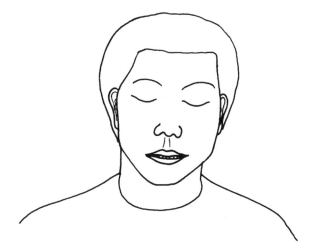

Fig. 3.40. Clicking the teeth together

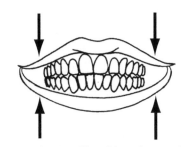

Fig. 3.41. Clenching the teeth

2. Close your mouth and let your teeth touch lightly. Direct your focus to your teeth. Gradually feel the electrical flow of energy there.

NECK MASSAGE

The neck is the busiest traffic site in the body. In addition to being the channel of the chi energy of the organs and the passageway for air and food, the neck is also the location of the thyroid and parathyroid glands (fig. 3.42), which regulate the body's metabolism and other functions.

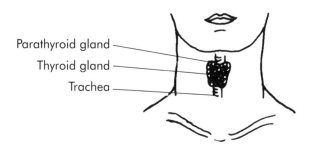

Parathyroid gland
Thyroid gland
Trachea

Fig. 3.42. Throat glands

Many meridians pass through the neck (see fig. 3.44 on page 56). In the middle is the Governor meridian. On each side are the Bladder meridian, the Gall Bladder meridian, the Triple Warmer meridian, and the Large Intestine meridian. Each of the meridians corresponds to certain emotions, as shown.

EMOTION	MERIDIAN/ASSOCIATED ORGAN
Anger	Liver/Gallbladder
Fear	Bladder/Kidneys
Grief	Large Intestine/Lungs
Hastiness	Heart/Small Intestine/Triple Warmer
Worry	Spleen/Stomach/Pancreas

Thus all of our emotions also pass through the neck. When we are under stress and emotional strain, the neck muscles unconsciously tighten, attempting to block out pain. This produces something like a traffic bottleneck in the neck. The emotions passing through the meridians of the neck become jammed. As tension in the neck accumulates, it interferes with the free flow of chi to all organs and parts of the body. Keeping the neck soft will help chi flow to the higher center that is located in the brain, keeping the mind and body in harmony together.

The neck also is the site of the power of speech, known as the Site of Courage. While tension in the neck can block self-expression and make us less courageous, the proper flow of chi energy through the neck fosters our ability to express ourselves appropriately at the proper time and place and in a proper way.

Performing Neck Massage

Begin with the procedure for bringing energy to the hands and contract the front of the anus.

1. Spread your thumbs apart from your other fingers. Alternating hands, rapidly wipe the neck from the chin to the base nine to thirty-six times (fig. 3.43).

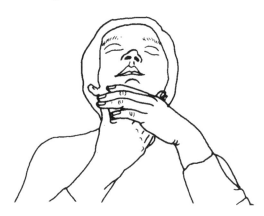

Fig. 3.43. Wiping the neck

2. Alternating hands, use the middle three fingers to rapidly wipe down the middle of the neck from the chin to the base nine to thirty-six times. The thyroid and parathyroid glands are in the front section of the neck. Use your thumb and the three other fingers to massage these glands. Find the painful points and massage them until you feel them open. Massaging this area will help to increase metabolism and the power of speaking.

3. Massage the points along the sides of the back of the neck (fig. 3.44). Use your fist to hit along the neck, starting from the shoulders and going up to the base of the skull (fig. 3.45). Find any painful or tense spots and massage until they are released. This will greatly help to release the tension of the neck and help to release the toxic accumulations in the neck area, the causes of many headaches.

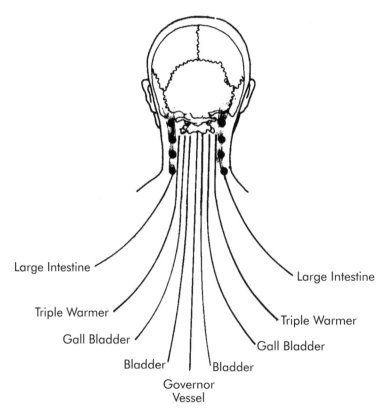

Large Intestine

Large Intestine

Triple Warmer

Triple Warmer

Gall Bladder

Gall Bladder

Bladder

Bladder

Governor
Vessel

Fig. 3.44. Neck meridians and points for massage

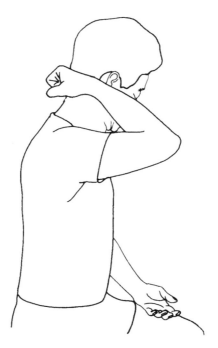

Fig. 3.45. Hitting the neck with the fist

Neck Exercises

1. Turtle Neck exercise: Sink your chin down, then out and up (fig. 3.46). Feel your spine press down and then expand. This will help loosen the vertebrae and discs of your neck.

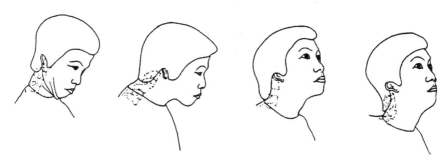

Fig. 3.46. Turtle Neck

2. Crane Neck exercise: Move your chin forward, circling out, then down, then up, and out again (fig. 3.47). Feel your spine expand and then contract.

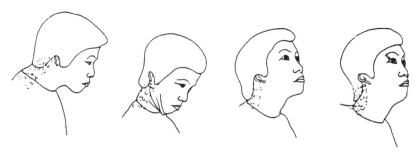

Fig. 3.47. Crane Neck

⚙ Shoulders Exercise

Many people feel tense and worried, and their shoulders are tight and held up. The tension can be released by doing this simple exercise.

1. Inhale as you pull up your shoulders to press against your neck, tightening the muscles of your neck and shoulders (fig. 3.48).

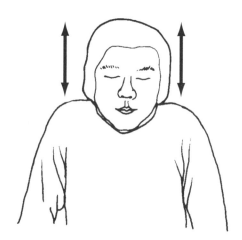

Fig. 3.48. Raising and lowering the shoulders

2. Hold for a while, exhale deeply, and let your shoulders drop down, pulled by gravity like a sack of potatoes. Feel the burden, worry, and stress drop down to your feet and out to the ground. Feel yourself grounded.

3. Repeat three to nine times, continuing to relax your shoulders and chest as you exhale and release the tension. The tension and worry will go away.

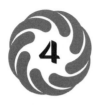

Detoxifying Organs and Glands

Toxic sediment can build up in our organs and glands, which interferes with their proper functioning and contributes to many health problems. Light slapping and tapping over the organs and glands releases the sediment and increases the circulation and chi flow to these areas, which helps to restore them. Our practitioners claim that they have been able to use this method to heal many chronic illnesses in themselves that conventional medicine had difficulty in healing. The slapping or tapping should of course be done in moderation, as excessive force can be harmful to the organs and glands.

MASSAGE OF
THE THYMUS GLAND

The thymus gland controls the immune system and is related to longevity. Normally the thymus gland atrophies after childhood. In the higher levels of Taoist practice, the thymus gland can be regrown, which helps to maintain health and vitality and supports greater spirituality. This massage of the thymus gland can help increase its activity and release more beneficial hormones.

Performing Massage of the Thymus Gland

Bring energy to your hands by the usual procedure, contracting the front of the anus and bringing the chi toward the thymus. Make a fist, inhale, and thump down the middle of the upper chest from the collar bone to the nipples six to nine times (fig. 4.1). Do not talk while you are doing this or you might harm yourself.

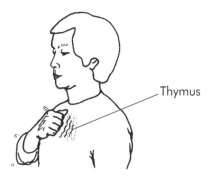

Fig. 4.1. Hitting the thymus gland

SLAPPING MASSAGE OF THE INTERNAL ORGANS

Lightly slapping the heart, lungs, liver, stomach, spleen, and pancreas stimulates the release of toxins, allowing the organs to rebuild and repair themselves.

Performing Heart Massage

Do the energy-to-hands procedure, contracting the left side of the anus and bringing chi toward the heart. Slap your heart lightly with your palm six to nine times (fig. 4.2). Don't speak while you are doing this.

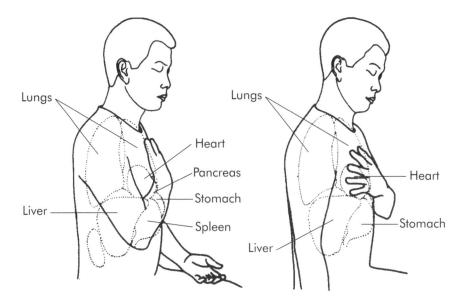

Fig. 4.2. Slapping heart, lungs, and liver areas

Performing Massage of the Lungs

Bring energy to your hands, contracting the right side of the anus and bringing chi to the lungs. Using your palm, slap up and down your right lung, hitting only as hard as is comfortable (fig. 4.2). Do not talk. Contract the left side of your anus and slap your left lung (fig. 4.2). This can help to clean out the mucus and to clear out the lungs.

Performing Liver Massage

Bring energy to the hands, contracting the right side of the anus and bringing chi to the liver (fig. 4.2). Using your palm, slap below the rib cage on the right side.

Performing Massage of the Stomach, Spleen, and Pancreas

Bring energy to your hands, contracting the middle and left side of the anus. Slap at the spleen, pancreas, and stomach (fig. 4.2). Then place one palm on top of the other and rub below the rib cage, from center to left, then left to center (figs. 4.3 and 4.4).

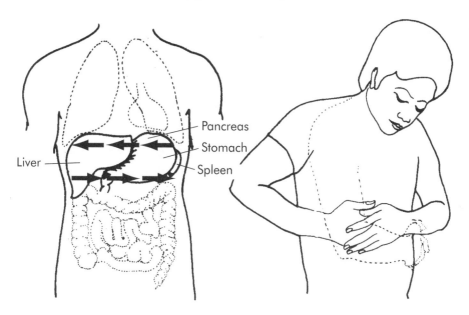

Fig. 4.3. Direction of forces for rubbing the liver, stomach, spleen, and pancreas

Fig. 4.4. Rubbing the liver, stomach, spleen, and pancreas

MASSAGING THE SMALL AND LARGE INTESTINES

A careless diet, such as one that contains too much hot food or dairy products or too little fibrous food, will create mucus that sticks to the walls of the intestines, which will block the absorption of nutrients and slow down digestion. Once mucus starts to accumulate, it is like a snowball that gets bigger and bigger, eventually becoming a lump that slows down the traffic of the digestive system, which can have many negative effects on overall health. Massage of the intestines increases absorption and dissolves the accumulations that stick to the intestinal walls. (Additional massage techniques for the intestines are given in the next chapter on relieving constipation.)

🌀 Performing Massage of the Intestines

Bring energy to the hands, contracting the entire anus.

1. Small intestine: With palms together, rub a small circle around your navel, first clockwise, then counterclockwise.
2. Large intestine: Place one palm on top of the other and rub your abdomen in a large circle. Start on the lower right side and rub up and around in a clockwise direction (figs. 4.5 and 4.6). This will move the energy in the intestine and relieve constipation. If you have diarrhea, rub counterclockwise. If you have normal elimination, rub in both directions.

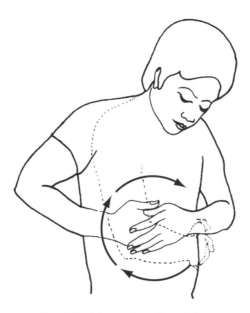

Fig. 4.5. Massaging the abdomen

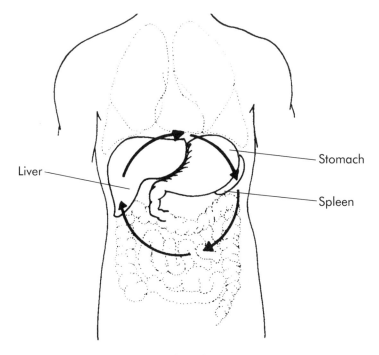

Fig. 4.6. Circling the energy

KIDNEY MASSAGE

The kidneys help to filter out waste material from the blood. If there is too much waste in the system, the kidneys cannot filter it all. The waste will tend to collect in the ducts and tubules of the kidneys, impairing their health. By hitting the area of the kidneys, we shake out the harmful sediment, crystals, and uric acid that get caught in the kidneys. This will strengthen the kidneys and help prevent kidney malfunction as well as relieving back pain.

 Performing Kidney Massage

Bring energy to the hands, contracting the left and right sides of the anus.

1. Locate the kidneys just above the lowest, or floating, rib in the back on either side of the spine. Make a fist and hit the kidneys with the back of the fist between the wrist and the knuckles (fig. 4.7). Hit only as hard as is comfortable.
2. Alternate hands and sides of the back.
3. Rub your hands together to warm them. Then rub your palms up and down over the kidneys until they feel warm.

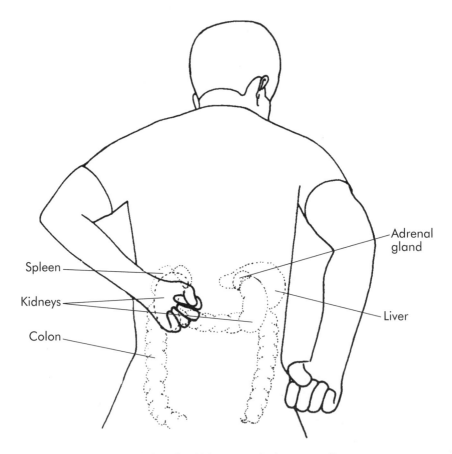

Fig. 4.7. Hitting the kidneys to shake out sediment

SACRUM MASSAGE

In the Taoist system the sacrum is regarded as extremely important. It is a pump that helps to bring spinal fluid and energy (chi) to the brain. It is also the junction where the sexual organs, rectum, and legs meet. Sciatic pain, which shoots down the legs, originates in the sacrum; therefore, strengthening the sacrum will relieve this intense pain.

 Performing Sacrum Massage

Bring energy to the hands, contracting the back of the anus toward the sacrum. Make a fist and use your knuckles alternately to hit both sides of the sacrum. Hit first in the area of the eight sacral holes and then the hiatus, the depression at the bottom of the sacrum (fig. 4.8).

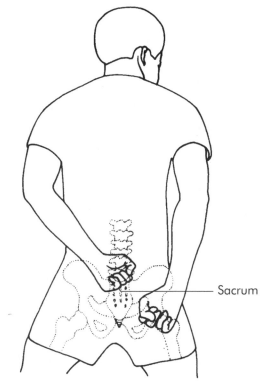

Sacrum

Fig. 4.8 Hitting the sacrum

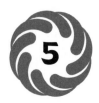

Relieving Constipation: A Major Cause of Ill Health

The key to good health is a clean colon. Conversely, constipation is a major cause of stress and disease. The modern life that we live—in the concrete jungle, where we eat refined foods, less fiber, more meat, and less fresh fruit and vegetables—causes us to have less chi. The pressure that moves the fluids and activates all systems in the body is weakened. This results in the stomach not having enough chi to digest food, the small intestine being slow in absorbing the nutrients, and the large intestine and rectum not having enough pressure to push the waste material out. When this material stays in the colon, the body reabsorbs toxins from the waste. These reabsorbed toxins first affect the liver. Next to be affected is the blood; as it becomes filled with waste material and toxins, the functions of other organs are disturbed, which lessens their ability to do their work and causes stress and nervousness.

Over time, the toxins that are retained collect throughout the body, causing it to age faster. For example, toxins in the skin make it coarse, not smooth; toxins in the neck and shoulder area result in headaches and shoulder pain. As they build up, these toxins can cause a hardening of the whole system. Constipation can lead to back pain, headache, stomachache, and colon cancer.

The effects are also felt emotionally. As the liver becomes filled with toxins, it produces negative emotions such as anger and anxiety. Long-term constipation can cause a person to become stingy and unable to let go of all kinds of unnecessary garbage. Keeping problems inside leads to overwrought emotions. The way to overcome this is to try to solve problems every day and speak out in a nice way, which will help the chi that is stuck in the organs to flow. However, speaking out in a way that is not nice causes more problems and more constipation.

Performing abdominal massage will help you to regain the nice feeling of a clean colon and a good flow of chi. That will help your whole day to be pleasant, open, and happy. It will foster the peace of mind that will permit you to solve problems in peace, letting you speak out in a nice way.

It is also important to go to the toilet whenever you first feel the need. Many people like to hold back until, after a while, the feeling of the need to move the bowel is gone. As a result, they have to hold it for the next time or the next day. It should become a habit to have a bowel movement every day; the morning is the best time.

ABDOMINAL MASSAGE: WONDER OF HEALING

Abdominal massage is one of the best ways to solve constipation. In the beginning you might see black and cloudy-colored bowel movements during elimination. This means that matter that has been stuck to the walls of the intestines for a long time has finally loosened.

You can do the abdominal massage right before you go to sleep and right after you get up. Usually shortly after doing this massage in the morning you will feel the need to go to the toilet to clear out the bowels.

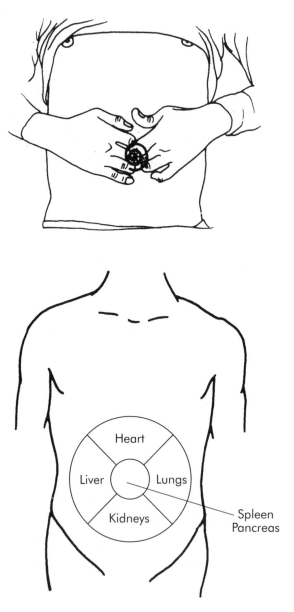

Fig. 5.1. Abdominal massage

🌀 Performing Abdominal Massage

1. Lie on your back, with your knees bent and your feet flat, shoulder-width apart.
2. Rub your hands until warm, then use your middle and index fingers to make small clockwise circles as you massage around the navel area (fig. 5.1).
3. Moving your index and middle fingers in small clockwise circles, massage the large intestine and rectum, starting from the lower end of the right side and moving up and across to the left side and down to the lower left side (fig. 5.2). Massage nine to eighteen times. Use your mind to help guide the chi flow according to the direction of the large intestine flow.

   If you feel a painful spot or a knot, spend some more time massaging there until it softens. It could be fecal matter that has

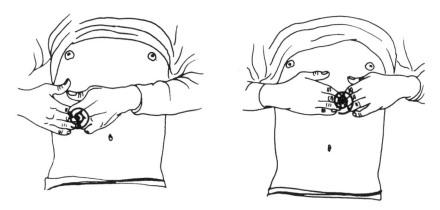

Fig. 5.2. Abdominal massage

hardened and remains stuck to the colon wall. People with weak energy who do not exercise the abdomen may not have enough energy to push fecal matter up the ascending colon or down to the rectum. Massage can break up the toxins and allow them to be eliminated.

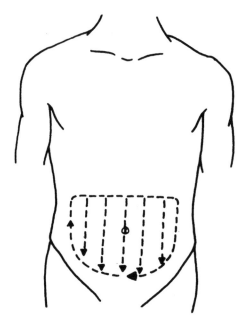

Fig. 5.3. Small intestine massage

4. To massage the small intestine, divide the abdomen into six parts (fig. 5.3). Using your middle and index fingers to make small circles, massage in a semicircle across the lower abdomen from the left line to the right line. Then continue making the small circular movements, following the pattern shown (fig. 5.3). Go up, down, and up each vertical line, then go to the next line. Repeat three to nine times. If you find a painful point or knot, massage clockwise and counterclockwise until it is gone. In the beginning you may feel like vomiting when you hit a painful spot. This is because the toxins are starting to clear out. Be cautious if you have had an abdominal operation; do only what is comfortable. If you feel pain in the area of the operation, rub it gently with your palm.

5. If you find a big lump while doing the massage at bedtime, put your palm over it and sleep with it there; this will soften the knot and release the pain and will help you to move your bowels more easily the next day.

✿ Massage during Bowel Movements

After you first move the bowels and stop and are waiting for the next movement, you can massage the abdomen to help clean out any "stew" that still is in the ascending colon.

1. Rub clockwise at the ileocecal valve at the right side near the hip bone. Massage from the lower end of the right corner up to the rib cage (fig. 5.4).

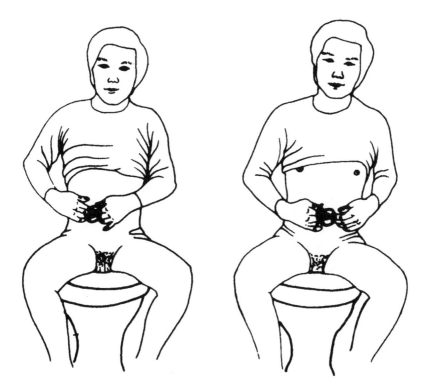

Fig. 5.4. Massage during bowel movements

2. Massage the sigmoid colon at the left side of the pelvis. Massaging this part can help you clear out more of the remaining "stew" (fig. 5.5).

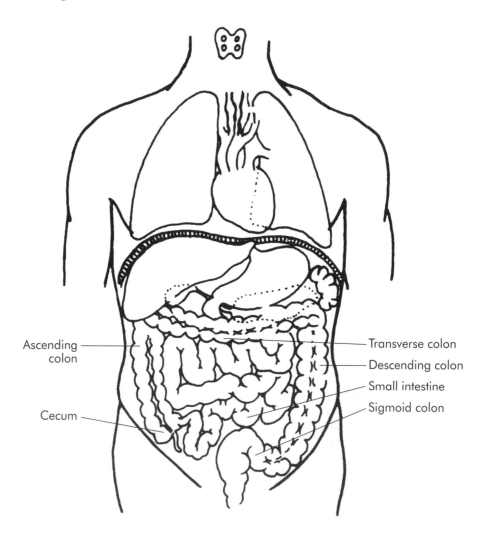

Ascending colon

Cecum

Transverse colon

Descending colon

Small intestine

Sigmoid colon

Fig. 5.5. The intestines and the sigmoid colon

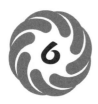

Knees and Feet

KNEE MASSAGE

Gravity has a slowing effect on circulation in the lower limbs, leading to the collection of toxins, particularly at the back of the knees. Slapping at the back of the knees will break down the toxins, allowing the body to eliminate them through the urine, bowel movements, and sweat. There is also very little blood flowing to the area of the kneecap and it tends to be quite vulnerable, which can contribute to a tendency to fall down. Massaging the knees will improve your stability and flexibility.

Performing Knee Massage

Begin as usual by bringing chi to your hands, with no contractions of the anus.

1. Bending over, or with your leg propped up on a chair or low table, and keeping your knee straight, slap smartly behind the knee nine to eighteen times (fig. 6.1). Although it hurts, this is an extremely effective way to release the toxins that have accumulated. This release may be indicated by the appearance of a purple dot. As with all Chi Self-Massage, be careful not to overdo it by slapping too hard. Repeat on the other knee.
2. Massage the right kneecap with the fingertips of both hands until it is warm, which will strengthen it. Massage the other kneecap.

3. Relax the kneecap, then move it up and down, to the left and right, and around both clockwise and counterclockwise (fig. 6.2). Repeat for the other kneecap.

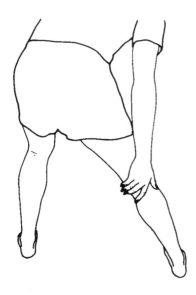

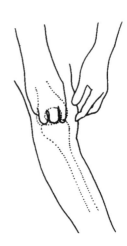

Fig. 6.1. Slapping behind the knee   Fig. 6.2. Massaging the kneecap

MASSAGE FOR THE FEET, THE ROOTS OF THE BODY

Strong feet and tendons increase your stability by connecting you to the healing energy of the earth. The feet are also like remote controls for the whole body, as the soles of the feet have energy meridians corresponding to all of the body's organs, glands, and limbs (fig. 6.3). Massaging the reflex areas on the feet will help to stimulate the corresponding organs and glands and increase circulation.

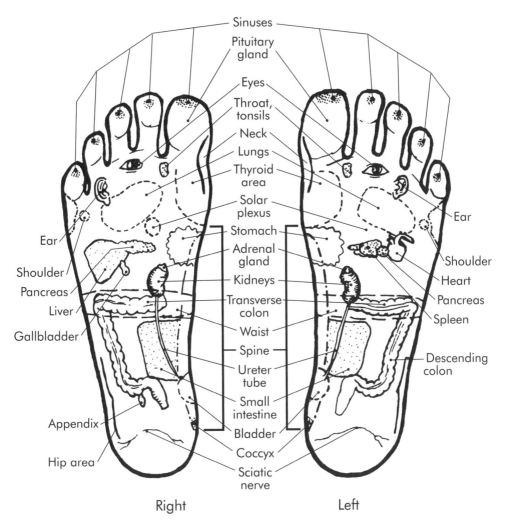

Sinuses
Pituitary gland
Eyes
Throat, tonsils
Neck
Lungs
Thyroid area
Solar plexus
Stomach
Adrenal gland
Kidneys
Transverse colon
Waist
Spine
Ureter tube
Small intestine
Bladder
Coccyx
Sciatic nerve

Ear
Shoulder
Pancreas
Liver
Gallbladder
Appendix
Hip area

Ear
Shoulder
Heart
Pancreas
Spleen
Descending colon

Right   Left

Fig. 6.3. Reflex areas on the feet

Performing Foot Massage

As usual, begin with bringing chi to your hands, with no contractions of the anus.

1. Take off your shoes and stockings and massage the tops and bottoms of each foot with your thumbs and fingers. When you find

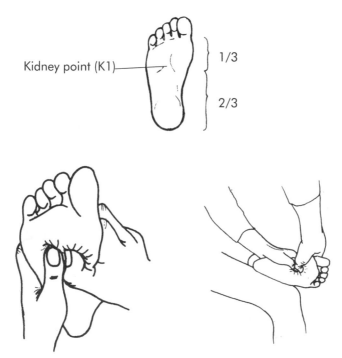

Kidney point (K1)

1/3

2/3

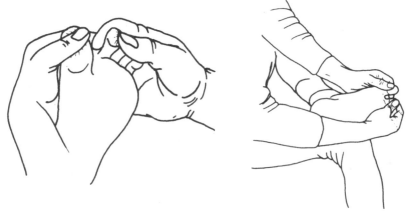

Fig. 6.4. Massaging the Kidney point (K1)

Fig. 6.5. Separating the toes

painful points, massage them until the pain goes away. This will help to clear any blockage of chi channel flow. Be sure to massage K1, the Kidney point known as Bubbling Springs, the sore spot in the center between the ball of each foot and the adjoining pad (fig. 6.4). If you are in a hurry, massage the whole of each foot once by rubbing the sole of one foot vigorously and carefully across the top of the other foot, going from the heel to the arch to the toes.

2. Spread out and separate all the toes, especially the little toes, and then release (fig. 6.5). Repeat six to nine times. This is especially good for the tendons of the feet.

3. Rub your feet together. This will help to keep the feet warm and will stimulate all the body's organs.

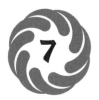

The Daily Practice of Taoist Rejuvenation

The goal of the Tao principle is to walk through to the end of life without sickness. In support of that goal, first-line prevention is best. Today huge parts of personal and national budgets are devoted to health care, and it has become very common for people to visit doctors and psychologists, go to hospitals, and even enter mental hospitals. An old man or old woman who is healthy and strong, able to walk and do things as he or she wishes, with no need to take pills and no use for Medicare, has become so unusual that the existence of such a person is often big news. But every one of us can be such a healthy old man or woman if we take care of ourselves.

The results of the Tao practice have been proven for many thousands of years. Tao masters have used it to maintain a high level of energy throughout the ages. This chapter presents the essential elements of Tao practice as daily routines that can be performed by everyone to support maximum physical and mental health. I encourage you to invest in your own health by making these routines as much a part of your everyday life as eating and brushing your teeth are now.

We all have the power to heal ourselves through transforming our negative emotions to positive emotions. But to get through negative states, you need to make up your own mind to set aside time and make this practice a part of your life. Don't worry about the results; simply keep practicing what you think is right for you. One day you will see the miracle happen. You will accomplish more work while becoming less emotional. You will seldom catch a cold and you will hardly remember your doctor's name. Your medicine box will be empty. You will be healthier than ever before.

Morning Warm-Up

If you have a good morning warm up, your whole day will run smoothly. The Taoist belief is that all organs have souls and spirits; when we are asleep, these souls and spirits are at rest too. They take a while to be awakened, and if we are too hasty, we can hurt them. So when you wake up, do not jump out of bed and do not open your eyes.

1. Open your heart first. The Taoist tradition says to open your heart before you open your eyes (fig. 7.1 on page 82). Imagine the heart as a red lotus flower. Inhale into the heart, drawing warmth from the sun; feel that warmth come down through the crown of the head and blend it with the chi in the red lotus of the heart. Feel how that energy circulates through all of your organs and limbs. As you exhale, imagine that energy carrying any accumulated toxins out of your system.

2. Warm your navel area. Without opening your eyes, put your palms on your navel area (fig. 7.2). Men, put your right palm on your navel with your left palm over it. Women, put your left palm over your navel and your right palm on top. Concentrate on your navel until you feel it become warm.

3. With your eyes still closed, do the Inner Smile energy practice (fig. 7.3) as instructed in the appendix. If you can, get in touch with the Inner Smile; feel the flow of it and guide the smile all the way down from the face to the neck and through the heart, lungs, liver, kidneys, pancreas, spleen, and sex organs. Smile into the digestive system and then the nervous system and spinal cord; sense when

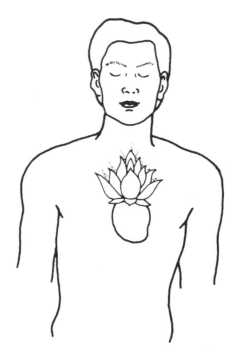

Fig. 7.1. Open your heart before your eyes

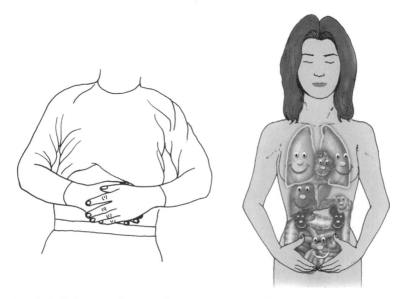

Fig. 7.2. Palms on the navel area   Fig. 7.3. Inner Smile

the smile can get through. Keep on smiling until any pain and tension go away.

4. Clear the energy blockages. We are all subject to natural influences that cause us to have cycles of high and low energy. If it is hard to get the smile energy flowing on a particular day, it indicates that your energy levels—physical, emotional, and intellectual—are at a low. Be very careful on such days, for when your energies are very low you are more likely to get into trouble and have accidents. However, by practicing the Inner Smile meditation, you can eventually overcome such cycles of low energy. If you smile through the organs and you feel obstructions and blockages in particular organs, take a little more time. Concentrate your awareness by smiling to that place where there is a blockage until it starts to clear up. When you feel your smiling energy increase and flow through the organs more quickly, that will indicate a raised energy level, which will give you more control over your emotions. This will help you to overcome or even avoid misfortune and accidents.

5. Do the Microcosmic Orbit meditation as explained in the appendix. Disease always begins with the blockage of energy flow to an organ or gland. When the major pathway to an organ or gland is blocked, the organ starts to get less energy, less blood flow, and less nutrition. When this persists over a long period of time, the organ or gland will work less effectively or not at all. No medical equipment or tests can check you out as accurately as your own awareness of your flow of chi. By the time doctors find an illness, an organ may be functioning at only ten percent efficiency. But doing a daily check-up on yourself using the Microcosmic Orbit meditation will enable you to correct, maintain, and strengthen yourself each day without spending much time.

6. Do the abdominal massage. The most important key to keeping healthy is to eliminate tension, worry, and toxins every day so that they do not accumulate in the body. Many people have great difficulty in getting up in the morning. They feel down, sluggish, and in a bad mood, with pain and aches all over. This is the result

of the accumulation of too many toxins in the body. The abdominal massage described in chapter 5 is the best way to clear out the toxins. Keep in mind that the abdominal massage and all aspects of Chi Self-Massage should begin with bringing energy to the hands, described in chapter 1, and at least a short hand massage, as described in chapter 2. Do as much abdominal massage as you can before rising and continue when you are at the toilet.

Increase Lower-Limb Circulation

When we are asleep, the circulation slows down, especially in the legs, which are the farthest away from the heart, and toxins start to settle in the legs and feet. Massaging your feet as part of your morning routine, following the instructions given in chapter 6, will help to clean out the accumulated toxins from the previous day and will stimulate the organs and glands. Including the following two exercises will add to the beneficial effect.

1. The Liver meridian runs through the outer corner of each toe, and the Spleen meridian runs through the inner corner (see fig. 7.9 on page 87). This exercise activates the liver, the major detoxifying organ, and boosts the immune system. Lying on a bed, rub the big toe and second toe of one foot back and forth against each other, twenty to thirty times, and feel the chi and circulation increase (fig. 7.4). Repeat for the other foot. This exercise can also help prevent hardening of the veins and arteries.

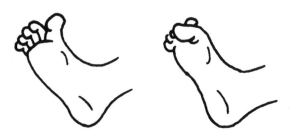

Fig. 7.4. Rubbing the toes together

2. Activate vein circulation. Veins are the return routes of the blood to the heart. Blood clots often occur in the veins of the feet, caused by high heels, tight shoes, or the wrong shoes, all of which tend to harden the veins and slow down circulation in the entire foot. The exercise is done by bending one foot at a time inward toward the stomach, while exerting force on the heel (fig. 7.5). Hold the position for a while and then relax. Men should begin with the right foot, women with the left. If your foot begins to cramp while doing this exercise, do not worry; simply use your fingers to pull your toes, bending them upward or downward until your foot recovers from the cramp.

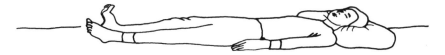

Fig. 7.5. Activating vein circulation

Morning Stretch Routines

When we are asleep, our tendons are at rest, not stretched out. When we get up, our body feels stiff and it is hard to move or bend. There are thousands of possible stretches that we can use to become more limber; we can spend a lot of time stretching. But if we do just a few stretches right, we can quickly stretch all the tendons and will not have to worry that we do not have enough time to start the day well.

When we feel stiff, hardening starts from the extremities. All the tendons and ligaments join together at the ends of the extremities: The feet, toes, hands, and fingers, as well as the tongue, which is the main connection place of all the tendons. Another area that may tighten is the spinal cord, with its connections of many tendons and ligaments. This set of stretches is designed to loosen up all of the extremities and the spinal cord.

1. Lying on your back, bend your back like a bow and stretch your hands and fingers while bending the feet toward the head (fig. 7.6). Spread and stretch out your fingers and toes as far as you can, then begin to do bellows-breathing: Exhale and suck in your stomach and abdominal area until it is flat and tucked in toward your spine, then inhale until that area is inflated. Repeat ten to fifteen times, gradually increasing the speed of your exhalations and inhalations.

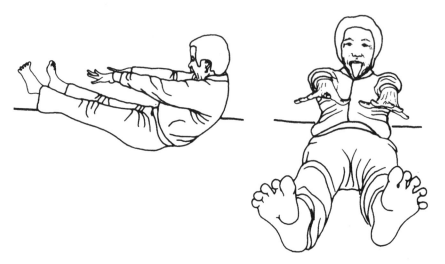

Fig. 7.6. Stretching the whole body

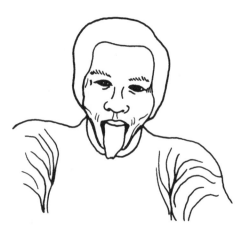

Fig. 7.7. Stretching the tongue

At the final exhale, exhale deeply and stretch out your tongue as far as you can toward your chin (fig. 7.7), while directing your eyes to look at the tip of your nose. Repeat this two or three times, then rest. The resting period is very important. Relax your body muscles totally and enjoy the flow of energy throughout your whole body.

2. From a sitting position, bend to touch your toes. Use your thumbs and index fingers to hold the big toes of both feet (fig. 7.8). This

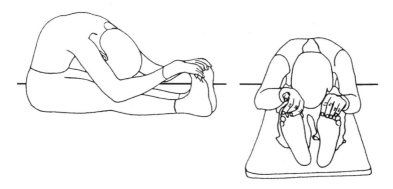

Fig. 7.8. Holding the big toes

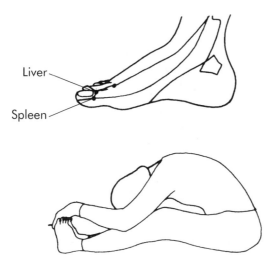

Fig. 7.9. Stretching the tendons

will energize the Liver and Spleen meridians (fig. 7.9). If you can't reach to your feet, reach as far as you can and hold the back of your knees or your calves. This will activate the Bladder, Lung, and

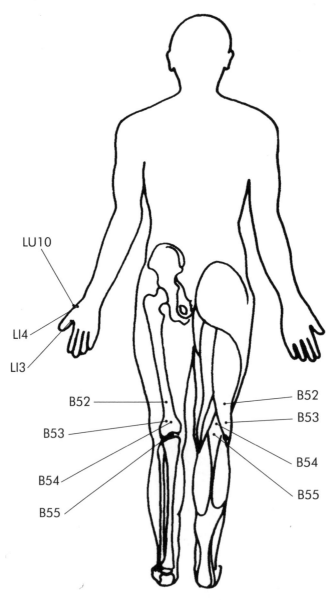

LU10

LI4

LI3

B52

B53

B54

B55

B52

B53

B54

B55

Fig. 7.10. Bladder, Lung, and Large Intestine meridian correspondences in the knees and hands

Large Intestine meridians (fig. 7.10). When your tendons are more stretched, you can move your hands to your ankles, through which the Bladder, Stomach, Liver, and Spleen meridians pass. Hold your ankles and feel the heat of your hands pass to the meridians. When you can stretch more, move to hold the toes and touch the K1 point to stimulate the Kidneys meridian.

Whether you are holding your knees, calves, ankles, or toes, begin to do bellows-breathing, starting slowly and gradually increasing until you feel your tendons and spinal cord get tense and then release. Once you feel the release, complete the bellows-breathing. After you finish, shake your feet and slap them a few times to loosen them.

3. To stretch out the neck and the spine, again bend over to touch your feet, but instead of bending your head toward your knees, look up and feel the stretching of your whole spine (fig. 7.11).

After doing these stretches, get up slowly. Roll your body slowly to the left side and sit up, then gradually stand up and walk.

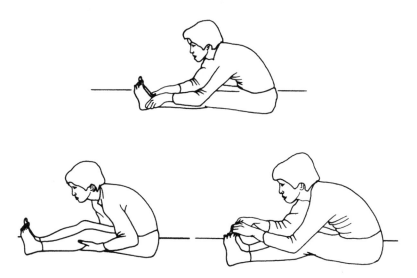

Fig. 7.11. Stretching the neck and spine tendons

CLEANING THE NINE OPENINGS

We have many openings in our bodies. Taoists say we have two doors and seven windows, which are the openings that permit us to have contact with the outside world. These openings are able to block out various kinds of pollution or let them enter. By keeping them clean and vital we help our whole body to be healthy.

Front Door: Sexual Opening

The sexual organ is regarded as the Front Door (or Gate), which is the door of the creative life-force energy. By knowing how to control and seal this door tight, the life-force energy will last longer. Men accomplish this by managing ejaculation, and women exert this control by conserving the energy normally lost to menstruation. These practices are explained in my Healing Love books.*

Back Door: Nutrients Opening

The anus is regarded as the Back Door (or Gate), which is related to nutrition. Many people are not aware of what to eat, so the body is unable to absorb the food being consumed. They end up losing most of the nutrients to their toilets.

In Tao we say that in order to keep the Back Door clean, you must first urinate, then have a bowel movement, then finish with more urination. Then use water to clean yourself. If this is inconvenient, use toilet paper that has been wet with water. The anus region has many arteries and veins, which clot easily and can become hemorrhoids. After cleaning, massage the whole region around the coccyx and the anus fifty to a hundred times. This is of great help in preventing or

---

Taoist Secrets of Love: Cultivating Male Sexual Energy (available through the Universal Tao Web site) and *Healing Love through the Tao: Cultivating Female Sexual Energy* (Destiny Books, 2005)

healing hemorrhoids, while helping to detoxify any accumulation in the lower region.

Seven Windows

The two eyes, two holes of the nose, one mouth, and two ears are the seven windows. We regard these windows as the openings of the organs:

- The eyes are the opening of the liver.
- The nose is the opening of the lungs.
- The mouth is the opening of the spleen.
- The ears are the opening of the kidneys.

The windows receive and transmit information, but if a window is dirty it will not receive information well; if a window is weak it will not adequately seal the life-force within. In order to maintain good health, daily maintenance is the best prevention. It is very important to use the Tao rejuvenation techniques given below to properly clean the windows each morning. Use the bathroom if you can, or another room if the bathroom is not available. You should also make the Chi Self-Massage techniques and exercises for the eyes, nose, mouth, and ears given in chapter 3 part of your daily routine, as time allows.

Eyes

Many times we do not pay much attention to the things that are closest to us, like water and air or our faces and eyes. Although most people wash their faces, they seldom wash their eyes. But in the course of the day, very small particles of dust and all kinds of fibers can get into the eyes and clog the tear ducts. So it is important to wash the eyes with cool, clean or boiled water.

Use a bowl in which you can immerse your face. Open your eyes and move your eyeballs around to get all the dirt and particles out

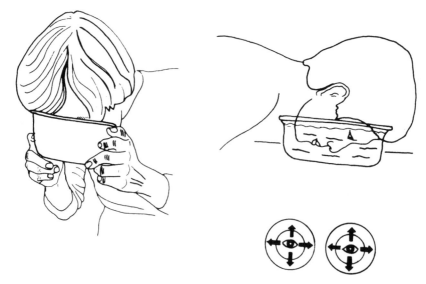

Fig. 7.12. Cleaning the eyes, nose, and face

(fig. 7.12). This will also help you to remain more awake. It is also important to massage and exercise the eyes as shown in chapter 3 (of all the exercises for the senses, the eye exercises are my favorite).

Nose

The nose is the place where the life-force of air enters. A strong and healthy nose is the key to vitality. Clean your nose right after you clean your eyes, using another bowl of clean water, preferably boiled water that has been cooled (fig. 7.12). Immerse your nose and face into the water, inhale a small amount of water into your nostrils, draw it up, then force it out through your mouth. In the beginning you might sniff or inhale too deeply and the water may go down your throat, which will cause you to cough. When you are well practiced, the water will smoothly enter your nose and come out of your mouth.

If you have difficulty handling both nostrils at one time, you can use your finger to close the right nostril while cleaning the left nostril, and then close the left nostril while cleaning the right. In the beginning you may feel pain or an unpleasant sensation, because the nose is like a chimney—if you never clean out the smoke, it will collect there. If you have time, also do the nose massage given in chapter 3.

Mouth

Weak gums are the cause of much tooth decay. Massaging the teeth and the gums with coarse salt is very useful for oral health. Using your index finger, touch the salt and then rub the inside and outside of your teeth and gums (fig. 7.13). Make sure that your finger is clean and the nail not too long. If you have time, also do the teeth and gum exercises given in chapter 3.

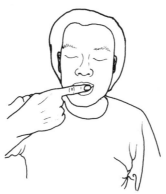

Fig. 7.13. Massaging with salt

The tongue is regarded as the opening of the heart. You should clean your tongue twice a day with a brush or scrape it with a tongue scraper. Massaging the tongue, as shown in chapter 3, is very important too.

Ears

Cleaning and massaging the ear shells and inner ears with a clean, damp towel will make you more alert and prevent hearing loss. Adding the outer and inner eardrum exercises given in chapter 3 will strengthen the ears.

USING THE MIRROR

We all use mirrors when we are combing our hair, and women often use mirrors to put on their makeup, but in Taoism we specially use mirrors to look at our own character and personality, and even the future. To foresee the future is not easy; it takes time to learn. We can more easily see how happy we are, physically and emotionally, and what is wrong with our organs and senses. Our face will reveal what is inside.

Look in the mirror at your face. Is it arrogant, angry, sad, depressed, or fearful? Try to change the expression to a happy, joyful, smiling face. Watch the corners of your mouth. If they droop down, massage them up. Do the face massage given in chapter 3 by first warming the hands and then massaging.

Your neck may reveal your age; a wrinkled neck might make you look old. Use a clean, damp towel and rub your neck until you feel the heat and chi flow in the neck.

Take time to massage your head as shown in chapter 3, and comb or brush your scalp carefully. This can be an enjoyable moment.

CLEAN WATER: WHOLE-SYSTEM CLEANSER

Water can help you clean out the dirt and toxins that remain in your digestive tract. Drinking two to four glasses of clean water in the morning, one to two hours before breakfast, is a very good way to clear out your system and provide prevention. Do not drink after a meal or before you sleep. If you drink at night, it will make you get up.

Boil the water if necessary to ensure that it is clean. Although at first it might be hard to drink a lot of water, you will slowly get used to it. After you drink, you need to move; you can walk, jog, or jump for some time. Then do the abdominal massage shown in chapter 5 to move the water around; it will rinse the toxins and mucus out of the body.

TAO REJUVENATION
THROUGHOUT THE DAY

The more you are able to do these Taoist practices, the greater the beneficial effect they will have on your health. Once you have learned the basic Tao rejuvenation routine given above, it should take only about ten minutes. To the extent possible, you should add to it as many aspects of Chi Self-Massage described in this book as you can. If you are rushed, try to do at least a few techniques, especially combing the scalp, getting a tear out, wiping the face and neck, hitting the thymus and kidneys, slapping behind the knees, and the foot massage.

You will discover that you will have many opportunities to fit these practices into your day. For example, you can do hand and finger massages while you are standing in line, waiting for people, sitting in a car, or reading a magazine or newspaper. You can do Chi Self-Massage while you are watching television.

Increasingly, more and more of our time is spent in transportation—cars, buses, airplanes, subways, trains, and so on—as well as waiting for transportation. You can use this time to do many of the self-massage techniques and exercises given in this book to refresh yourself. However, if you are driving, be very careful; use your own good judgment. Do not do any exercise that will disturb your vision or attention on the road.

 Commuting Exercises

Here are some additional exercises that can be done while you are commuting:

- The neck is usually the most tense and can cause nervous tension. To loosen it, do the shoulder exercise given in chapter 3, inhaling as you pull your shoulders up to press into the sides of the neck and then pull your scapulae together in your back; tense the spine and scapular muscles for only a few seconds, then exhale and drop your shoulders.

- It is important to keep your spine loose and relaxed so that the chi can flow without obstruction. To aid this, hold your seat with your hands, pull your stomach in toward your spine, and imitate a "bowl," with your chin touching your chest and your pelvis and sacrum tucked in. Tense the back muscles for a few seconds, especially the muscles around the kidneys, and then release; you will feel nice fresh energy rise to the top of your body and circulate down the front.
- Sitting on both of your hands, palms up, will give your whole body a general revitalization. You will be able to feel the chi from the palms and fingers steam up through your bottom to the base of your spine, helping you to feel refreshed in a short time.

Relief for Stress and Fatigue

These techniques can help with the tensions and stress of modern life, whether on the job, while commuting, or in other situations that may arise.

- Holding the fingers, as shown in chapter 2, will help you rid yourself of negative emotions such as worry, fear, and anger.
- When you feel dull or sleepy or cannot think right, cleaning the teeth and clicking the teeth together as described in chapter 3 will be extremely helpful in clearing your mind.
- When you feel tired or fatigued, contract the left and right sides of the anus as shown in chapter 1 and wrap the

chi around the kidneys. You will help to increase the kidneys' capacity to clean out the toxins and give you more life-force energy. Contract the right side of the anus to stimulate the liver. This will help give you vitality and the ability to make decisions more easily. Contract both sides of the anus and wrap the chi around the lungs. In general, pulling up the different parts of the anus will stimulate the corresponding organs, as described in chapter 1.

- If you feel sleepy while driving a car, use the following techniques, which are sure to keep you from falling asleep: the clicking-teeth exercise; moving your shoulders up to tighten your neck and then releasing them; pulling up the anus to vitalize the kidneys; and using your pinky finger to hold the steering wheel tight to increase circulation.

- If you work sitting at a desk or at a computer for long periods of time, it is very important to exercise your eyes, neck, and kidneys. Every one to two hours, close your eyes, massage your eyeballs, and move them around until you feel good. Another excellent exercise is to periodically hit the kidney and sacrum areas, as shown in chapter 4. If you can also take ten minutes to do the Inner Smile, the results of your work will improve (any company that gives its employees time to do these practices will surely benefit).

ENDING THE DAY

Evening Practice

In the evening before you go to bed, find time to soak your feet in hot water for five to ten minutes and wipe them dry. Rub them until they are hot, and do each of the Six Healing Sounds three times, according to the sequence described in *Taoist Cosmic Healing*.

Sleep

How we sleep is also important to our health. Do not wear tight clothes. Choose a good pillow: one that supports the neck, rather than one that supports just the head, leaving the neck hanging high in the middle. Flowers in the sleeping room can help you to sleep well, but do not use overly fragrant ones because they can cause you to have a lot of dreams. If you feel constipated, do some abdominal massage for a while before sleeping.

Give care to your sleeping position:

a. If you like to lie on your back, lie with your arms and legs straight, and lightly hold your thumbs in your fingers (fig. 7.14a).

b. If you sleep on your side, try to sleep on your right side with your spine straight, your left leg bent, your right leg straight, your right hand's palm on your head but not covering your ear, and your left hand on your hip (fig. 7.14b).

c. You can also lie on your side with your spine straight, curving your two legs in, and put both hands between the legs (fig. 7.14c).

"OH, NO! NOT ANOTHER OBLIGATION!"

The crux of any self-improvement program is continued practice. Of course, it takes a certain amount of inner discipline to practice the techniques in this book on a regular basis, preferably every day. Yet a basic tenet of Taoism is flexibility, accommodation to natural circumstances. So be flexible with your rejuvenation program; make it suit your individual schedule. Do as much of the routines as you have time for. If you have time only for the Lung and Kidney sounds, do just those (but not before bedtime, as they are energizing when done individually). If you have only two minutes for the Inner Smile, do a quick "waterfall of smiling energy" through your body.

Most important, try to integrate the practices into your daily life, smiling down whenever you think of it and doing the Healing Sounds

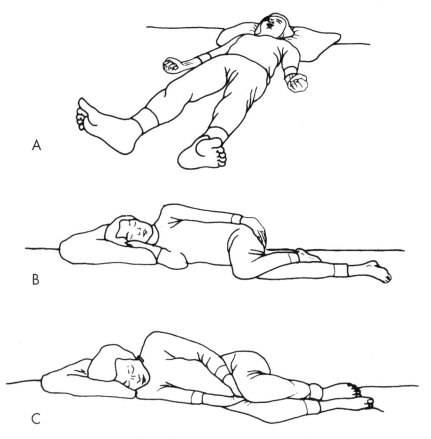

Fig. 7.14. Sleeping positions

when you need to relax, to deal with a particular symptom, or before bedtime. Use the eye exercises after reading, writing, or other close work. Get rid of a headache by doing the crown exercise, the temple massage, and bridge-of-the-nose pinching.

Chi Self-Massage and all of the other practices of Tao rejuvenation are marvelous tools for relaxation and well-being, not another burdensome task to feel resentful or guilty about. Play with them and use your creativity to incorporate them into your personal lifestyle. Make them yours. Enjoy feeling, looking, and functioning as a happier, calmer, more vital, and more attractive person.

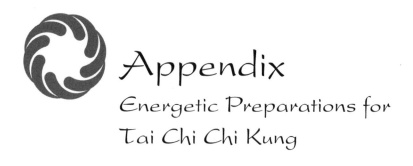

Appendix
Energetic Preparations for Tai Chi Chi Kung

INNER SMILE

The Inner Smile is a powerful relaxation and self-healing technique that uses the energy of happiness and love as a language to communicate with the internal organs of the body. A genuine smile transmits loving energy that has the power to calm, balance, and heal.

When you smile inwardly to the organs and glands, your whole body feels loved and appreciated. The Inner Smile begins at the eyes and mid-eyebrow point. The eyes are connected to the autonomic nervous system, which in turn is connected to all the muscles, organs, and glands. As one of the first parts of the body to receive signals, the eyes cause the organs and glands to accelerate activity at times of stress or danger and to slow down when a crisis has passed. When the eyes relax, they activate the parasympathetic nervous system and cause the rest of the body to relax.

As you activate the loving energy, you will feel the energy of the Inner Smile flow down the entire length of the body like a waterfall. This is a very powerful and effective tool to counteract stress and tension.

There are three vital aspects to each phase of the Inner Smile. First, direct the awareness to a specific part of the body. Second, smile to that part of the body; send it a genuine feeling of love, gratitude, and appreciation for its role in keeping the body running smoothly and in good health. Third, feel that part of the body relax and smile back to you.

❧ The Inner Smile Practice

1. Stand in the Wu Chi stance or sit on the edge of a chair with the hands comfortably clasped together and resting on the lap. Keep the eyes closed and breathe normally. Follow the breathing until it becomes smooth, quiet, deep, even, calm, and soft.

2. Relax the forehead. Imagine yourself in one of your favorite beautiful places in the world. Recall the sights, sounds, and sensations of that place until they are vividly in your mind's eye. Then imagine suddenly meeting someone you love. Picture him or her smiling lovingly and radiantly at you. Feel yourself basking in the warmth of that smile like sunshine, drawing it into your eyes. Feel the eyes relaxing and responding with a smile of their own.

3. Picture the healing chi of nature—the fresh energy of waterfalls, mountains, and oceans—as a golden cloud of benevolent loving energy in front of you. We call this the Higher Human Plane energy of the atmosphere, the blended chi of heaven and earth, or the Cosmic Particle force. Direct the smiling energy in the eyes to this Cosmic Particle energy around you, drawing it into the mid-eyebrow point. Feel the brow relaxing and widening. Spiral the energy into the mid-eyebrow point; feel it amplifying the power of your smile.

4. Let the smiling awareness flow down over the cheeks, down through the jaw muscles and tongue, and down through the neck and throat, soothing and relaxing as it goes.

5. Smile down to the thymus gland and the heart. Feel them open like flowers in the morning with love, joy, and happiness bubbling out of them.

6. Smile down to the rest of the solid organs: lungs, liver, pancreas, spleen, kidneys, sexual organs, and reproductive system. Thank each of them for their work in keeping you vibrant and healthy. This completes the first line of the Inner Smile.

7. Return your awareness to your eyes and recharge the energy of

your smile. Then draw in more of the golden light of the Cosmic Particle force.

8. Roll the tongue around the mouth until you have gathered some saliva. Smile to the saliva and draw the smiling energy and the golden light into the saliva, transforming it into a healing nectar.

9. Swallow the saliva in two or three strong gulps. Follow it with awareness down the esophagus, smiling as it goes, feeling the healing nectar soothing and refreshing the esophagus. Continue smiling through the rest of the digestive tract: the stomach, small intestine, gallbladder, large intestine, rectum, anus, bladder, and urethra. Thank these organs for their work in giving you energy through ingestion, digestion, absorption, and elimination. This completes the second or middle line of the Inner Smile.

10. Return your awareness to your eyes and recharge your smile. Then once again connect with the golden light of the Cosmic Particle force.

11. Now smile to the brain, to the left and right hemispheres, and to the pituitary, thalamus, and pineal glands. Then smile down through the spinal column vertebra by vertebra, thanking each vertebra for its work in protecting the spinal cord and supporting the skeletal structure. This completes the third or back line of the Inner Smile.

12. Return your awareness to your eyes once again and recharge your smiling energy.

13. Smile down through the whole body, particularly to any place that feels tired, sore, painful, weak, empty, or tense. Shower these parts with the healing nectar of your smiling awareness.

14. Finally, smile to the navel and collect the energy there.

15. Starting in the center of the navel, begin spiraling the energy outward. Men should spiral the energy in a clockwise direction, making thirty-six revolutions; women should spiral the energy in a counterclockwise direction, also making thirty-six revolutions. Take care not to make the outer ring of the spiral any larger than a grapefruit; circling above the diaphragm causes too much energy

to flow into the heart and overstimulates the emotions, and circling below the pubic bone sends too much energy into the reproductive system, where it may be lost through ejaculation or menses. After completing the first set of revolutions, spiral inward in the opposite direction twenty-four times, ending at the center of the navel.

MICROCOSMIC ORBIT MEDITATION

The Microcosmic Orbit meditation awakens, circulates, and directs chi through the Governor Channel, which ascends from the base of the spine to the crown, and the Functional Channel (also called the Conception Vessel), which runs down the front midline of the body. Dedicated practice of this ancient esoteric method eliminates stress and nervous tension, energizes the internal organs, restores health to damaged tissues, and establishes a peaceful sense of well-being.

The meditations of the Microcosmic Orbit system also strengthen the Original Chi and teach you the basics of circulating chi. They allow the palms, the soles of the feet, the mid-eyebrow point, and the crown to open. These specific locations are the major points at which energy can be absorbed, condensed, and transformed into fresh new life-force.

The Tai Chi classics say, "The mind moves and the chi follows." When you focus your attention at a specific place in the body, you automatically activate the chi at that place. By the mere act of attention, you consciously link the brain to the local sensory receptors at that place. The nervous system in turn creates local changes in capillary circulation, muscle activity, and lymphatic flow.

All the movements in these systems require energy; we call this energy chi. The sensations of these energetic changes can be subtle or dramatic. They are characterized by such feelings as warmth, tingling, pulsing, expansion, vibration, and effervescence. You may sense one or more of these feelings depending on your level of sensitivity and your experience with meditation and Chi Kung. Don't worry if you feel little or nothing at first; just focus your attention at each point.

Whether you feel it or not, your chi will be moving. With practice, you will begin to feel the chi moving more vividly.

Spend at least one to two weeks concentrating on completing the Microcosmic Orbit before proceeding to learn the Tai Chi Chi Kung form. Read through the books *Awaken Healing Energy through the Tao* and *Awaken Healing Light of the Tao,* paying special attention to the question-and-answer sections.

Basic Microcosmic Orbit Meditation Practice

1. Begin your meditation practice with the Inner Smile. As you did for the Inner Smile, stand in the Wu Chi stance or sit on the edge of a chair with your hands comfortably clasped together and resting on the lap. Keep the eyes closed and breathe normally. Follow the breathing until it becomes smooth, quiet, deep, even, calm, and soft. Smile down to the front, middle, and back lines to relax and harmonize the body, breath, and mind. Then smile to the lower tan tien, but do not collect energy yet.

2. Activate the Original Chi in the lower tan tien. Focus your attention on the tan tien, breathing naturally using lower abdominal breathing. Use your intention to create a feeling of warmth in the lower tan tien. Feel it as the reservoir of your Original Chi, the main battery of your entire energetic system. Imagine that each breath is like a bellows fanning the fire in the lower tan tien. Hold your awareness there until you feel the lower tan tien is filled with chi.

3. Begin to move the energy in the Functional Channel. Move the awareness to the navel and concentrate there until you feel the energy has gathered at that point. Then bring the attention to the sexual center (Sperm/Ovary Palace). When you feel sufficient energy gathered there, proceed in a similar way to the perineum (Gate of Life and Death).

4. Direct the energy through the Governor Channel. When you have accumulated substantial energy at each point, move the awareness to the next successive point. From the perineum, continue concentrating the energy at each point up the spine to the head: to the coccyx, the sacral hiatus, the Door of Life, T11, the Jade Pillow, the crown, and the mid-eyebrow point (the third eye).

5. Now connect the two channels. Bring the attention to the tip of the tongue. Touch the tip of the tongue to the palate, connecting the two main channels of the Microcosmic Orbit. Press and release the tongue against the palate nine to thirty-six times. This activates the palate point and enables the energy to flow down the Functional Channel.

6. Complete the circulation in the Functional Channel. Direct the attention to each point along the Functional Channel: to the throat center, the heart center, and the solar plexus and back to the navel. This completes one cycle of the Microcosmic Orbit. You may notice less sensation in the Functional Channel because there are seven parallel pathways along which the energy may descend, and thus the energy may become more diffuse.

7. Continue to circulate energy through the Microcosmic Orbit. Circulate energy through the entire cycle at least nine times. As you gain experience you can increase the number of circulations to 36, 72, 108, or 360. At some point you may feel the energy begin to move by itself. This is a good sign. If it happens, don't try to restrain it; just let it flow at its own pace.

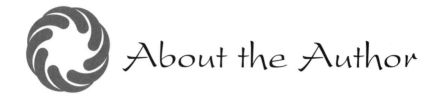 *About the Author*

Mantak Chia has been studying the Taoist approach to life since childhood. His mastery of this ancient knowledge, enhanced by his study of other disciplines, has resulted in the development of the Universal Tao System, which is now being taught throughout the world.

Mantak Chia was born in Thailand to Chinese parents in 1944. When he was six years old, he learned from Buddhist monks how to sit and "still the mind." While in grammar school, he learned traditional Thai boxing, and he soon went on to acquire considerable skill in aikido, yoga, and tai chi. His studies of the Taoist way of life began in earnest when he was a student in Hong Kong, ultimately leading to his mastery of a wide variety of esoteric disciplines. To better understand the mechanisms behind healing energy, he also studied Western anatomy and medical sciences.

Master Chia has taught his system of healing and energizing practices to tens of thousands of students and has trained more than two thousand instructors and practitioners throughout the world. He has established centers for Taoist study and training in many countries around the globe. In June 1990 he was honored by the International Congress of Chinese Medicine and Qi Gong (Chi Kung), which named him the Qi Gong Master of the Year.

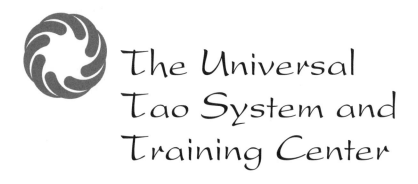

The Universal Tao System and Training Center

THE UNIVERSAL TAO SYSTEM

The ultimate goal of Taoist practice is to transcend physical boundaries through the development of the soul and the spirit within the human. That is also the guiding principle behind the Universal Tao, a practical system of self-development that enables individuals to complete the harmonious evolution of their physical, mental, and spiritual bodies. Through a series of ancient Chinese meditative and internal energy exercises, the practitioner learns to increase physical energy, release tension, improve health, practice self-defense, and gain the ability to heal oneself and others. In the process of creating a solid foundation of health and well-being in the physical body, the practitioner also creates the basis for developing his or her spiritual potential by learning to tap into the natural energies of the sun, moon, earth, stars, and other environmental forces.

The Universal Tao practices are derived from ancient techniques rooted in the processes of nature. They have been gathered and integrated into a coherent, accessible system for well-being that works directly with the life-force, or chi, that flows through the meridian system of the body.

Master Chia has spent years developing and perfecting techniques for teaching these traditional practices to students around the world through ongoing classes, workshops, private instruction, and healing sessions, as well as books and video and audio products. Further information can be obtained at www.universal-tao.com.

THE UNIVERSAL TAO TRAINING CENTER

The Tao Garden Health Spa and Resort in northern Thailand is the home of Master Chia and serves as the worldwide headquarters for Universal Tao activities. This integrated wellness, holistic health, and training center is situated on eighty acres surrounded by the beautiful Himalayan foothills near the historic walled city of Chiang Mai. The serene setting includes flower and herb gardens ideal for meditation, open-air pavilions for practicing Chi Kung, and a health and fitness spa.

The Center offers classes year-round, as well as summer and winter retreats. It can accommodate two hundred students, and group leasing can be arranged. For more information, you may fax the Center at (66) (53) 495-852 or e-mail universaltao@universal-tao.com.

For information worldwide on courses, books, products, and other resources, contact:
Universal Healing Tao Center
274 Moo 7, Luang Nua, Doi Saket, Chiang Mai, 50220 Thailand
Tel: (66)(53) 495-596 Fax: (66)(53) 495-852
E-mail: universaltao@universal-tao.com
Web site: www.universal-tao.com

For information on retreats and the health spa, contact:
Tao Garden Health Spa & Resort
E-mail: info@tao-garden.com, taogarden@hotmail.com
Web site: www.tao-garden.com

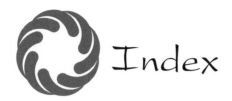

Index

Page numbers in italics refer to illustrations.

BOOKS OF RELATED INTEREST

Tan Tien Chi Kung
Foundational Exercises for Empty Force and
Perineum Power
by Mantak Chia

Healing Light of the Tao
Foundational Practices to Awaken Chi Energy
by Mantak Chia

The Inner Smile
Increasing Chi through the Cultivation of Joy
by Mantak Chia

Wisdom Chi Kung
Practices for Enlivening the Brain with Chi Energy
by Mantak Chia

Chi Nei Tsang
Chi Massage for the Vital Organs
by Mantak Chia

Energy Balance through the Tao
Exercises for Cultivating Yin Energy
by Mantak Chia

Iron Shirt Chi Kung
by Mantak Chia

The Secret Teachings of the Tao Te Ching
by Mantak Chia and Tao Huang

Inner Traditions • Bear & Company
P.O. Box 388
Rochester, VT 05767
1-800-246-8648
www.InnerTraditions.com

Or contact your local bookseller